Surpassing the Shame

on Being Gay, Bipolar, HIV-Positive, and Addicted

Surpassing the Shame
on Being Gay, Bipolar, HIV-Positive, and Addicted

Insights from the Client and His Therapist

Daniel P. Kennedy and
Kathy Vader, M.A., Theology and Psychology,
Licensed Psychologist

2017
FuzionPress
Burnsville, MN

Copyright © 2017 by Daniel P. Kennedy and Kathy Vader

All rights reserved
Printed in the United States

No part of this book may be reproduced in any form whatsoever without permission in writing from the authors, except by a reviewer, who may quote brief passages in critical articles or reviews.

First Printing 2017
20 19 18 17 16 5 4 3 2 1

ISBN: 978-1-946195-16-6

Library of Congress: 2017948600

FuzionPress
Burnsville, MN
FuzionPrint.com

Edited by Connie Anderson, Words & Deeds, Inc.
Interior Design by Sue Stein

Names and places were changed to protect the privacy of those mentioned—and all references are to "he," even though a large number of women deal with the same issues as Daniel does.

This book was written over almost a decade, and the authors decided to use present tense in the areas written in the earlier years—so we can understand how the author felt when it happened.

All prescription drugs that are brand names will appear with a ® only the first time mentioned. (See list end of book.)

*To my parents whose love gave me life, and my husband,
Brian Garland, whose life gives me love.*
—Daniel

Advance Praise for *Surpassing the Shame*

This book is a "must read" for anyone who has loved a person diagnosed with bipolar disorder. Growing up as a child in the 1970s with a mother who was undiagnosed until the early 1980s was often very scary. My mother was frequently angry and clearly ashamed of the highs and lows that ruled her life, which left my father, my sister and me feeling hurt by her actions—and guilty that we could not help her.

After reading Daniel's story, I have found peace and a deeper understanding of my mother's struggle. The medical care and counseling that have enabled Daniel to persevere through adversity to lead a happy, "normal" life, simply were not available to my mother as she was subjected to experimental drugs, treatments and little-to-no counseling. Daniel's story has helped me to understand how hard my mother tried to be a good parent—and to appreciate her strength and courage as she struggled throughout most of her adult life with a condition that no one acknowledged or understood.

—*Jeanne Lynch Babula, high school teacher*

Not only did the book deliver a strong, clear message, but I felt that it went beyond its stated purpose of helping bipolar individuals and their loved ones. As a total layman in the field of psychology, I early on began to develop a connection with Daniel as I followed him through his personal battle. I felt that I was living his struggle with him, and though I have in reality been free of the symptoms he fought, I gained a new understanding of them. It was if I was drawn into his world, although at the outset, it was completely foreign to me. For a "mainstream" guy like me to strike a chord with a man like Daniel, dealing with the complex issues he faces, testifies to the clarity of this book.

Because Daniel and Kathy wrote with such emotion, such frankness and such clarity, I see the book as having wide appeal far beyond the community of the diagnosed and their therapists. Any layperson with even an ounce of curiosity about bipolar, HIV, chemical dependency, and the impact of any or all of these on a gay man can gain important insight from this book.

But sympathy was my overriding emotion the more I came to know Daniel. I feel that lack of understanding on the part of society as whole with respect to the issues Daniel faces is what prompts anger and blame toward individuals like him. To a large extent, he has had to fight his battles in the darkness of his own mind, and it has been only through the help of an amazingly insightful therapist, a loving husband, and a supportive family that he has been able to find the light at the end of the proverbial tunnel. And he was blessed with his doctor and therapist who never gave up on him.

The important message that *Surpassing the Shame* delivers—sometimes graphically and shockingly; sometimes tenderly and with great caring—is that we must continue to further our understanding of these disorders.

—*John Shepard, layperson, parent and grandparent, and 1957 Stanford graduate*

Daniel Kennedy has presented an honest and thought-provoking portrayal of his life with bipolar. As his father, this was certainly not easy reading, but then again, nothing about bipolar is easy.

Surpassing the Shame brought me moments of discovery and revelation, fury and heartbreak, and finally, pride and hope. The trip that Daniel and Kathy take you on will allow you to see the challenges of living with bipolar, and show you that this condition *does not* preclude a happy and productive life.

If you are trying to understand and help a loved one with bipolar disorder, this book will give you some very valuable tools.

—*Ed Kennedy, Daniel's father*

This is an important and well-written book about an individual who is challenged by his sexual orientation, a diagnosis of bipolar disorder, multiple health issues including HIV, and his chemical abuse/addiction. It addresses the complexities of these issues and the role played by the client's feelings of shame, guilt, fear, anxiety, depression, and self-defeating behaviors.

Daniel's writings clearly show the importance of his motivation to change, his honesty, and his strong relationship with his therapist—and to her patience and skills. Readers will gain great insight into human behavior from both the client's and therapist's perspective.

This book is humanistic, insightful, thought provoking, empathetic, sensitive, informative, and helpful. It is of benefit to individuals who are struggling with these issues or anyone who wants or needs a better understanding of them.

—*Gary A. Malkes, B.A., M.S., LISW (Retired);*
worked with juvenile sex offenders

Table of Contents

	Foreword	1
1	My First Manic Episode–Age 18	3
2	Therapy: All Roads Lead Somewhere	9
3	Acknowledging Being Gay—and Diagnosis of Bipolar	17
4	Encountering Abusive Men in Gay Lifestyle	23
5	Detour on Road to Marrying Mason	29
6	My Husband Insists I Enter Treatment	39
7	My Treatment Program—and Sober-house Living	45
8	HIV-positive and a New Therapist	57
9	Depression, Mania, and Medication	73
10	Religion and Spirituality	79
11	Watching His Words	85
12	Let's Talk About Sex, Shall We?	93
13	The Letting-Go Process	99
14	Shame-Based Feelings	109
15	Meeting Brian Garland, the Love of My Life	117
16	The Two Ends of the Co-Dependence Continuum	123
17	The "Bipolar Curse"	133
18	Personality Type to Understand Yourself	139
19	Extremes of Bipolar Disorder: Rage and Shame	147
20	The Black Hole of Depression	155
21	Mania Is More…	161
22	The 12-step Program: Daniel's Point of View	171
23	What is the Harm-Reduction Model?	191
24	Spirituality and Addiction…and Masturbation	199
25	Medications for Bipolar and HIV	209
26	Correlation Between What We Put into Our Body—and How It Functions	213

27	"Living" on Welfare Payments	229
28	Importance of Trust and Acceptance in Your Life	237
29	Moving Far Away to "Back Home"	245
30	Myths and False Beliefs	257
	Important Points to Remember	259
	About the Authors	263
	Reading Resource List	267
	Acknowledgments	273
	Addendums for Therapists	277
	List of Prescription Drugs/Brand Names	287

Foreword

Shame is a debilitating experience when it is a result of an attack on the very being of a person. Anyone who has been shamed for some aspect of "self," such as enduring a mental illness, being gay, or suffering from an addiction, knows this. In my practice, a person living in shame has a difficult time loving himself. And that shame ripples through every aspect of that person's life, including work and relationships. Daniel's story is a testament to this.

Surpassing the Shame is a deeply personal story of one man's struggle with being gay and feeling different, discovering he is bi-polar, and to medicate his shame and depression, he turned to chemical use. Luckily, Daniel found the therapist, Kathy, who was right for him, and in her humanistic approach, she demonstrated unconditional acceptance and compassion. This engendered a therapeutic relationship built on trust that was so necessary to Daniel's healing. Treating body, mind, and spirit all at the same time was a challenge, but eventually led to Daniel not giving up and even finding self-love, so necessary to healing any shame.

Daniel and his therapist tell the story from their unique perspectives, giving the reader the opportunity to understand the complexity of living with a bi-polar diagnosis and its challenges in treatment. It also points out the relationship between shame, trauma, addiction, and a bi-polar diagnosis. Learning about the emotional losses and financial cost of these illnesses will hopefully help a person develop empathy for those they live with and love who struggle with shame, bi-polar illness, or addiction.

As a psychologist and addiction specialist, I believe that if a person could wish these problems away, they would do so in a heartbeat. The adage, "Pull yourself up by your bootstraps" is not only impossible in such situations, it shows little understanding of those who suffer. But shame almost kept Daniel from seeking the help from Kathy that was needed—and changed his life forever.

—Brenda Schaeffer
Licensed Psychologist and Certified Addiction Specialist
Bestselling author of *Is It Love or Is It Addiction?* and *Love's Way*

Chapter 1

My First Manic Episode—Age 18

At the age of eighteen, and in the fall 1998 semester at college, some two hundred miles from home, I had my first severe manic episode. I will never forget the details. With several days of being awake behind me, my mind could not calm its own thoughts. More and more time passed without sleep. The lack of calm in both mind and body led to utter and total exhaustion. My thoughts turned more and more erratic and dangerous. I recall seeing what I perceived as demons flying around, and to escape them, I spent the better part of one night running up and down the ten flights of stairs in my dorm building, dehydrated and completely drained, and slipping deeper and deeper into the terrors of insanity. At last, the bottled-up energy pierced the vessel of my mind, shattering the glass like a Molotov cocktail. In October of the fall semester I received the diagnosis of bipolar disorder, and was put on lithium. It is important to note that my first psychiatrist gave me *no real information*—only a prescription and an order for lab tests every three months.

As devastating as the diagnosis was, I did not understand what I was facing and what I had to live with every day. The lithium caused me to start putting on a lot of weight. I began feeling lethargic all the time, as well as disconnected from my surroundings. For some people this simple salt compound corrects the bipolar disorder very well, but not for me. For me it just made a bad situation worse. I was still very uncomfortable with my diagnosis, and was fearful of what people would think of me if they were to know. At this time the circle of people who knew was limited to close family and personal friends.

Time passed, and when I went back for the second semester, mania hit me, and it hit hard. I didn't need sleep, I stopped eating and started acting extremely irrational, and without any limitations. For the first few days I was elated. I believed I could do anything. To people around me at school, it seemed I was in an incredibly good mood. I thought the work I was getting done was so brilliant, but in truth, it was incomprehensible and erratic. After a few days, my mood turned from elated to wrathful. I began tearing apart everyone and everything in my path, screaming like a madman at my roommate, being nasty to my friends, and even getting mouthy with professors. By day five, I was ripe with sheer rage, formed by the swirl of emotions moving through my head at light speed. This time, as would happen many times, I lashed out at the person to whom I felt the closest, in this case, my mother. When I called home, I went on a verbal tirade. I spoke of my disdain for God and Catholicism. I ripped at every fiber of my belief system that I could relate to my mother, and lashed out at her value system.

I was in such agony that my only relief seemed to come from spitting my venom like a King Cobra ready to devour its prey. For what seemed like an eternity, I struck out, over and over again, physically damaging the objects in the room around me, and verbally abusing this mother of mine. During this episode I had one underlying hope—I could drive the wedge far enough into our relationship so my mother would stop loving me. Then I could die without a single strain of guilt on my remaining and deteriorating conscience, and maybe, just maybe, I could find peace. The end goal never did surface this night. A few days later, and after many concerned phone calls from home, my father came to see me. I can only assume he was terrified of what he would find. He even told me he was going to "be in the area," so I wasn't defensive or closed to his visit. The manic episode had broken, and I was in a deep and severe depression. Suicidal thoughts were present in their horrifying glory, and I was drained of all hope of ever feeling anything but misery. This is frequently the case with bipolar depression.

Hours later, I was headed home with my father, having dropped out of college. I was now starting down the early bricks of my very own road to a rainbow. But a rainbow can come only if there is rain.

Moving to California

My parents agreed to send me across the country to live with my aunt and uncle who had experience dealing with mental illness, and bipolar disorder. The idea to do this actually came from my aunt who has lived with bipolar disorder her whole life. Her children also dealt with mental health issues, and at the time they were really the most trustworthy and knowledgeable resources that any of us had to turn to on a personal level. I started therapy for the first time while living in California, and although I saw that therapist for only nine months, it was my introduction to the benefits therapy could have.

But usually, when manic, there was, there is, this rage. Anger is a very common emotion a person with bipolar disorder taps into when he's cycling. Sometimes it is simply the anger of having to deal with a brain that, if you'll forgive the pun, has a mind of its own. Chemical emotions and receptors in the brain are wildly fluctuating, and without knowing what is happening, you have the danger of acting out of total impulse, doing and saying things that are both dangerous and frightening. A complicating factor was that I had never learned how to properly express normal anger, so multiply a normal feeling of anger a thousand times over, and you get a vortex of rage, without any boundaries or the caution of rational thought. As these manic episodes continued into my twenties and thirties, the focus of the rage, once directed at others, managed to merge with my shame, and the new victim of my punishing mania *became me*.

I turned into a self-destructive force hell-bent on crucifying myself over and over in a multitude of ways.

A desire that feels primal in this state of mind caused great harm to me and to all I hold sacred. This mania has led to my being raped at a sex club; willingly being infected with HIV; multiple years of drug use, usually stimulants and whatever else I could get my hands on. I smoked, snorted, and injected crystal meth, crack cocaine, powder cocaine, heroin, ketamine,

GHB, and I am sure a litany of substances I don't remember. I became what addicts often refer to as "a garbage can," meaning if a drug was available, I used it. Imagine referring to oneself as a garbage can. The self-loathing is often so well portrayed in the verbiage used to describe it.

Mania led me to cheat on lovers, steal from strangers, shoplift, drive with no concern for others on the road, and put myself in mortal danger. This must be horrifying to read because it is horrifying to write, I assure you. I think it is important to state that for many years I believed I had no control over my behavior when I was manic. I thought through a lens of hopelessness, I could do my best only when I was in a place of stability. During depressions I am often left almost paralyzed, and during mania I am a destroyer. This left only the times of remission available for my own genuine self to live and thrive until I was able to learn how to navigate the episodes. Unfortunately I needed to address so much damage in between episodes, even those stable moments were lost to recovering from the damage.

It would take a lot of time and more work than I ever thought I had the capacity to do in therapy to finally come to believe, in fact, I was not powerless over this illness.

Yes, sometimes I cannot overcome the depression, and have to work with managing my medications, and push through to the other side. Other times when I am manic, I still have the impulse to do drugs, to hurt myself, and to attack the things I love in my life because I don't think I deserve them. Having said this…

- If I utilize the resources at my disposal, I am able to navigate both depression and mania to sounder seas,
- If I get in touch with my psychiatrist when I feel an episode coming on,
- If I keep up with my therapy sessions so I have a constant gauge of whether or not I am high or low,
- If I eat healthy foods, natural and whole foods, and take my medication as prescribed,

- If I choose to stay active and not be sedentary.

Choosing to eat healthy foods and use them as fuel, and to exercise *in whatever ways I can sustain,* I can navigate my bipolar episodes in a way that's not horrifying and destructive. I am still struggling with my own laziness in this area.

It is hard work, and I cannot ever let down my guard, but I am emphatically telling you it's absolutely worth every ounce of energy I put into it. I can always do something else to get through the hard times. I am not a scary person living a scary life anymore,

- I am stable and have a sound mind that sometimes has to be rested or eased, which I am able to do through talking and dispelling the shame.
- I do it by learning how to properly express my anger when I feel it, and not allow it to fester like a sore that won't heal.
- I do it by accepting that everything that has happened to me in life is an opportunity to learn and grow.
- I do it by forgiving others for falling short and being human, and forgiving myself for the same things.

If we are not willing to show compassion to ourselves, how can we ever truly empathize with others, and show them the compassion this world so desperately needs.

Now I get it—I deserve happiness and compassion.

Bipolar disorder is not my fault, and it doesn't have to be my identity. It doesn't have to be yours either, but you have to be willing to work hard and learn as much as you can as you go. If someone in your life wants to truly love you, he or she will also learn about it. I have lost friends and relationships because of ignorance, which is a true loss to all parties. You might find people are afraid of your mental illness. Encouraging them to learn about it dispels the fear, and in the long run, helps you. Bipolar disorder has taught me that life is ready to offer us what we need if we are willing to also give others what they need. It's balance, and even in the world of extremes that is bipolar disorder, there can be achievable balance, a life living with the illness as a part of it, but not controlling it.

Chapter 2

Therapy: All Roads Lead Somewhere

> *therapy (n.) 1846, "medical treatment of disease," from Modern Latin therapia, from Greek therapeia "curing, healing," from therapeuein" to cure, treat medically, literally "attend, do service, take care of;" related to, therapon "servant, attendant."*
>
> —www.etymonline.com

How can the term, so ubiquitous in popular culture, which describes something so healthy and positive, also continue to be associated with stigma and fear? I suppose it is not at all surprising in a society that rewards false perfection, and persecutes the real weaknesses and challenges that make us human. After fifteen years of therapy, I am certain it is the single most effective tool of self-discovery I have ever encountered. Its forms are vast and its uses range from overcoming psychological scars to simply having a safe place to meditate about one's own life and values. But therapy is more than just a tool in our healthcare workshop. Therapy can represent a commitment to oneself to help enlighten the soul and validate the great benefits of human imperfection. It also embodies our desire to improve (not to perfect) our lives—to accept ourselves and others both as we are and as we have the potential to become through self-discovery, self-destruction, and self-(re)creation.

Therapy is a garden of change where the cultivation of meaning-making and care of the self can achieve full bloom.

My diagnosis of bipolar disorder type 1 brought me to therapy. I had no idea it would do so, but it has cemented in me the truth that my life is *about my choices*. It continues to give me peace surrounding my decisions, actions and reactions, along with the understanding that I choose my own perspective. I cannot always choose how to feel, but I can choose how I cope with and respond to these feelings. This choice helps me to create a reality I can truly own.

A couple of the most common stigmas about being in therapy describe it as a place to go complain and whine—or that it is only for people who struggle with a serious mental illness. In reality, it is a place where personal responsibility is embraced over all else. My time in therapy has spanned many different professionals in the mental and somatic (body) health fields: psychiatrists, psychologists, general practitioners, electroconvulsive therapy specialists, cardiac care doctors, and internists.

What psychotropic medications do to the human body biochemically can often be as dangerous as the mental health illnesses the drugs are designed to treat, causing a need to find medical professionals who can truly attend to the entire person. A psychotropic drug is simply any drug that directly impacts a person's mental state, and as you will soon read, I have been on a gaggle of these drugs. Some have worked well; others have not. Mostly, the meds I take do a fairly good job of controlling my symptoms, at least enough to help me function in the day-to-day life I choose to live. Of course there is a trade-off that comes in the form of side effects and damage that these medications do to my body and how it functions. I will go into greater detail about all of that later. For now let me focus on the different forms of therapy I have embraced in my life. I sought counsel from priests, friends, and community leaders. I had at times expected family members and 12-step sponsors to be my professional voices of guidance. These expectations were totally unrealistic and unfair, and they have often led me into dangerous situations, and influenced me to make dangerous mistakes. I have disagreed with doctors who were unwilling to consider any treatment other than ones with which they were comfortable, and have also tried numerous alternative therapies: nutritional supplements, Reiki, meditation, acupuncture; the list is seemingly endless. Nevertheless, there has been value in all of it. The positive experiences have helped me learn more about myself biologically, psychologically, spiritually, and emotionally. The negative experiences have taught me more about what works for my biology, my psyche, and my own chemical health.

Of all the tools I have had at my disposal, none have been more challenging or more liberating in my quest for quality mental and overall health than the therapeutic process itself. A person needs to attend to all areas of life—the numerous needs of the whole person. At this point in my journey, it is my firm belief that I seek balance and validation more than anything else, and the therapeutic process is the greatest tool at my disposal as I strive to be the healthiest and most contented self I can be. Too often, people stop having therapy after one bad experience. This is completely understandable, given the enormous challenge of feeling so vulnerable while simultaneously having to become one's own complete advocate. We need total honesty, not just for ourselves, but with the therapist in order to work through whatever the challenges may be. Yet our shaping experiences, and the inability to sometimes trust our own minds, let alone another person's, are always there trying to steer us off course. It is most important to be able to embrace and accept the complex spectrum of possible colors in a world bent on spreading the simplistic delusions of black and white. A world where there is one absolute truth is often fatal to those who suffer through the torment of the mind. As there is not just one kind of client in the world, there is not *only one* type of therapist, one psychiatrist, one path to God, or one personality. Every person may find his own strength to embrace who he is, and accept what works best for his own personal value system congruent with his own personal understanding of what "healthy" is or can become.

Although I believe my bipolar disorder symptoms began around the age of ten as I entered adolescence, it was not until the age of eighteen when I was finally given a diagnosis, or had I sought any type of professional help.

High school was tumultuous to say the least. I was struggling not only with this unacknowledged mental illness in addition to all the usual dilemmas of teen life, but also the reality of being gay, closeted, and also devoutly Catholic, which can be something of a quagmire. There was little support to ease me through the fears of both issues, and I did not see any way to reconcile the impasse. This was not anyone's fault. These were the cards dealt to me, and learning to play my own hand has always been the backbone of developing who I was, am, and will become.

I was not at all popular in my school years. It seemed that I was always frightened. I was scared to answer questions in class for fear of being wrong, and thus not look intelligent. I struggled to relate to my peers who seemed to have interests that were not at all similar to mine. While I did not have a lot of bullying directed specifically at me, I did not fit anywhere. I always seemed to be older than I was intellectually, and I was certainly emotionally more complicated than most of my classmates.

My saving grace in those high school years, before I knew that I was living with bipolar disorder, ended up being the special teachers that I encountered. There was a spirituality teacher who I really admired. He engaged me in the one subject I was passionate about at that time—religion, and the questioning of the universe around me, and my purpose in it. I was close to my bus driver and to a couple of other random teachers. The most supportive was Jeanne, my algebra and chemistry teacher. When I met her, she was in her mid-thirties. Every day I anxiously waited for the time I was able to spend in her class. She identified me as "struggling" very early on, and she devoted a lot of time and consideration to my continued growth and success as a student and as a person. When I was around her, I felt like I was actually being heard. I would often spend time after school in her classroom studying or getting extra help.

Academically I was much more talented than I was ever able to express. Every day I had an impossible time sorting through the myriad of emotions that were ever-changing, and opening up to Jeanne about the things I was thinking and feeling, would gave me a sounding board that quite literally saved my life. More days than not, during those teen years in the mid 1990s,

I pondered suicide, or fantasized about just disappearing from life altogether. I was repressing my sexuality so vehemently, and was turning to all the wrong places for help. Jeanne knew I was gay long before I was able to admit it to myself or anyone else. She went to bat for me with other teachers when I struggled to apply myself to my studies, and she always had time to talk to and listen to me.

To Jeanne, I was not an outcast or just another student. She helped me to rally and get through the entire four years. To this day Jeanne and I are friends, and the relationship means the world to me. I needed someone to stand up for me and notice that I was in agonizing mental pain all the time—and Jeanne did. So, when I look back on my high school experience, it is not the classes or the friends I had that resonate in my memories. I remember the lessons of how to be resilient and steadfast. I remember learning how to never give up, even in the face of total despair. I was learning that even when I did not feel a part of the larger community, or sense that I had anything in common with any of the other students, I was going to be okay someday, as long as I kept fighting to learn, grow, and survive.

A truly remarkable teacher is someone who can sense when a student is in trouble, and knows instinctually how to reach out to that person and offer compassion and a place to belong. I did not have any level of understanding about the challenges I was facing mentally or spiritually, but I was being taught how to survive and persevere until I could one day understand *who I was*, and how I could successfully navigate the experience of being true to myself.

During adolescence, the only person I was consciously aware of suffering from bipolar disorder was a distant cousin who, while off his medication, stabbed a police officer in my hometown. How could I face my own mental illness when this was my strongest image of it? Homosexuality was still stigmatized in every outlet of my life as *abnormal* in the least—and a mortal sin at most. What teenager wants to be abnormal? I suppose many can and do thrive on that—but my dream was to fit in, and be accepted. As for sin, my belief at the time was that I was a mortal sinner, and if I acted or even explored my feelings about my sexuality, I would be banished to an eternity in hell.

As it turned out, the only hell I had to worry about was the one I was creating with my shame and silence. I come from a family whose core belief is love, but a lack of exposure to and knowledge of mental health and sexuality issues made it very difficult for me to be honest with myself, or to ask for help. So I turned to the only resource I knew at the time: religion. Religion is not a bad thing, and I harbor only gratitude for the tremendous upbringing I had at home, and in the Catholic Church. I am no longer a Catholic, but I do have a well-defined sense of my spiritual self, and find great solace and sometimes, great challenges on my spiritual journey.

For the most part, the friends and acquaintances that have filled my life have also been connected to some sense of spirit, and I have learned great things sharing spiritual experiences with others, even when those experiences have greatly differed from my own. Today I am writing this as a secure, proud, gay man who understands what my sexuality means to me. But at the time, being gay was terrifying. Visions of sugarplum fairies were, well, just that. I had no reason to believe I could be who I was—and be gay. In the world and at the time I grew up, it meant I was a sexual deviant, who, since I was gay, would obviously become a pedophile, and would fill the world with disease, and tear at the very fabric of society.

Where all these beliefs came from doesn't matter. Repressing something innately true about oneself is as damaging to one's mind and soul as anything could possibly be. It is so easy in hindsight to place blame on why and how one's belief system was formed. For a long time, I chose to blame my family for not fostering my gay self. I could choose to blame a two-thousand-year-old religion for not yet being ready to change its teachings on homosexuality, even though overt expressions of modern gay identities in mainstream culture were still in their infancies.

There have always been and will always be homosexuals. We are everywhere. However, we *are not* all unnatural predators or deviants. We are simply people, who, for whatever reason, are naturally attracted to people of the same gender. A culture has formed around us, and stereotypes often do fit, but not those of criminality, malice, and sin. I have encountered deviance and predation among fellow homosexuals, but gays certainly have no monopoly—evil is human—*and it is a choice.*

> Gay-dar—intuitively knowing someone is gay—because of exaggerated gestures, words/voice, clothing, sensibility, flamboyance, as well as a fluid subversion of traditional gender roles, including hyper-masculinity and exaggerated femininity, as well as devotions to fashion, aesthetics, melodrama and Broadway—many of these stereotypes flourish in the diverse lesbian, gay, bisexual and transgender (LGBT) community, but seldom in one personality.

I did not fit into any of the traditional gender roles, and my personality has always been more feminine than masculine. I'm a feeler first; everything else comes second for me.

Cultural stereotypes of any variety or association form usually out of some snippet of truth, which doesn't mean they speak holistically as truth. Maybe they offer a way to laugh about the frequent absurdity of the human experience. People of all races and backgrounds, beliefs and circumstances, deserve to be respected as human beings. Absurdity can unite us, even as a mark of difference. Accountability for one's actions is not sacrificed when acceptance of one's reality is achieved.

During my time as a nursing assistant in my early twenties, I worked with patients who had Alzheimer's disease and dementia. A trick I learned has proven invaluable in my quest for my own mental health. If you try to force someone out of her reality and into yours, she will fight it with every fiber of her being. However, if you can be wise and patient enough to meet someone where she is at in her own reality, she will feel respected and validated, and more times than not, she will be willing to accept your reality, even if she doesn't agree with it. I could not tell an Alzheimer's patient I was not her late husband, and I could not force other people who were new to the reality of my being both gay and struggling with mental illness, to accept these essential but challenging facts. How could I, when I was terrified of *accepting my own reality*.

Wisdom and understanding come only from time and process. Redemption, also in the secular sense, stems from devastation. One must grieve any loss before accepting the gifts to be gained from it. To let go, sacrifice and surrender something valued and precious, in exchange for something else unknown, we have to first feel safe. Otherwise, we birth resentments and ignorance, coupled with a superhuman desire to hold onto what we already know.

> **One must grieve any loss before accepting the gifts to be gained from it.**

Chapter 3

Acknowledging Being Gay—and Diagnosed as Bipolar

I was raised in Rhode Island on the East Coast. My world changed at the ages of eighteen to nineteen when I lived briefly with extended family in California. It was there that I first saw a psychotherapist. I was newly diagnosed as bipolar, and for many reasons it was easier for me to begin the process of coping with this new diagnosis in California than where I grew up. When I left California in November of 1999 and returned to the East Coast to try to reclaim my life, I had the subconscious awareness that I was going to have to find my own way—but subconscious knowledge was only a start. There was so much I had not learned, about my mental illness, what it meant to be a gay man, and at only nineteen, what it meant to be human. I left thinking I was "cured," when in actuality I had only scraped the surface of some very challenging truths about myself.

After I moved back in with my parents, I began experimenting with sex. My confused thought process was that if I were going to go forward with embracing *my true self*, including my sexuality, I would have to let go of the idea of waiting to be married to experiment sexually. Same-sex marriage was not even on anyone's radar yet, neither the public's nor mine. I was coming to terms with the teachings of my religion. The truth was, and this is what I perceived—*I was going to go to hell because of my homosexuality.*

So what good was it to wait for love or marriage to express my deeply repressed sexual desires?

I dated women, but had no sexual relationship with them. I had sex with men, but a relationship was not a concept I could yet fathom. I decided to lose my virginity to a stranger, which seemed an easier way to cope. Soon I was having more and more sex with more and more strangers—and I was not protecting myself, physically or emotionally.

My first medication therapy was lithium. Lithium carbonate is a salt that is used as a common treatment for bipolar disorder. For some it is a miracle cure, but it never had a positive effect on me. Back on the East Coast and now on meds, I had not continued on with the therapy process. Doing so would have been tremendously helpful for me to cope with the next three years, but at the time, I thought therapy was just for sick people, *and I was "cured."*

The lithium was not controlling my bipolar disorder, but I was still years away from being able to tell the difference between my moods and feelings. I just figured taking the medication meant that I was fine. It became clear with time that I was not fine. It was then that we added a medication called Depakote to the mix. Depakote is a seizure medication that has proven helpful with mood stabilization, and as a treatment for mania in people with bipolar disorder. Over the next few months, I saw no change in my moods. In fact the only thing this drug did was to damage my liver. I could not metabolize the medications I was on. My cholesterol was skyrocketing, along with my blood pressure. I gained weight at what felt like a pound a day. At six feet tall, I have always been a big guy—but now I was pushing 250 pounds. My color was off and, along with my moods, my energy was swirling further and further down, like flushing a toilet.

This was my emotional state when I decided to come off of my medication, and this time also corresponded with my decision to lose my virginity to that first stranger. If the medications were not working, my thinking was it might not be bipolar disorder. Maybe it was time to come out of the closet. So, in my typical fashion, I dove out of the closet, balls to the wall, and into a big pool of glitter. My personality is boisterous to begin with. Add a few manic episodes, and it can really be a spectacle to behold.

I bleached my hair to platinum blonde, bought and wore only the shiniest and most extravagant clothes. I became the caricatured stereotype I had in my mind of what a gay man was. It was time to try it out, so I turned to the only place I realized existed at the time to meet other men like me—the internet, another amazing tool, but it can be oh so very dark if misused.

I found a man online I was willing to have sex with, or rather who I thought was willing to have sex with me. His name was Dave, or so he said. He instructed me to rent a motel room, and he would meet me there. I arrived an hour early, rented the room, and then drove around the block for at least forty-five minutes. I did not want someone I knew to spot my car parked there. Finally I got the courage to go to the room and wait for this man. When he arrived, I found myself ready to vomit from nerves, and learned for the first time what I would come to learn again and again.

People can pretend to be anything they want on the internet as a way to achieve their desired goal. Translation: this "Dave" was not a nice man, nor had he posted an accurate picture online, but rather some likeness of a self he may have been twenty years earlier. His stated age of thirty was a lie of at least a decade, and he stank of booze and smoke. But, there he was, and I felt somewhere inside that "it was now or never."

The entire experience took all of six minutes. He treated me as an object, and used me with force. I let him do it, although it hurt in ways I had never experienced. No tenderness, no love, no unifying experience, just a sketchy middle-aged man using me. His violent thrusting made me scream into the pillow, and when he left the room, he threw twenty dollars on the nightstand as his "contribution" to the cost of the room.

For a while, I stayed in this sty of a room, hurting all over, and crying, wondering why anyone would believe in a God of love. Was it all a joke? Perhaps the polytheism of Greek mythology was the real truth. Zeus and his friends were all up there pushing us around like pawns on a chessboard, showing favor to the few, while laughing at the agony of the many. And if creation were to be believed, why would God create sex, and then make some people desire this type of sex? From my limited experience, I guessed that being in a successful gay relationship must mean one party is hurt and abused by the other.

I was never more wrong about anything, but for the next several years it was exactly what I thought, and it was fueled by my deteriorating mental health, and my warped views of what it was to be a gay man. Medications came and went, as did psychiatrists. I began the difficult process of going against everything I had ever believed in spiritually, and drama was the air I breathed.

Being in crisis became my strength. I jumped from job to job, person to person. My boyfriends were all abusive in one form or another. Some were physically forceful with me, while others brought me to sexual places where I was not comfortable. More often than not, I became totally dependent on having a boyfriend, any boyfriend. If someone was willing to date me, this translated in my mind as being of value as a person. I did not matter how bad the abuse, or how big a loser he was, in my mind I was not a "victim," I was a willing participant in it all.

This is where my friend Kate comes into the story. Kate was an acquaintance from high school, and I enjoyed her company. So, when I was twenty-three I called her and asked her if she was interested in finding an apartment together. This is bipolar thinking at its most classic, calling someone out of the blue that you haven't seen or talked to in a few years, and asking them to move in with you. At the time Kate said "no," but it was the seed of a friendship the likes of which I had no idea I would come to rely upon so heavily.

It is so very important to realize mental health is sort of a dichotomy. It can be all consuming without the proper help, and even sometimes with all the available help being utilized. It can take all of your attention and energy. At the same time, to be healthy everything has to be in balance. This means having a therapist, psychiatrist, and doctors who I trust—those who work with me, and do not try to impose their beliefs and pictures of health onto me. It also means having an active spiritual life, a sense of purpose, and solid, intimate relationships.

I have many tremendous friendships in my life, and many of them have turned into members of what is often referred to in LGBT communities as "family of choice," meaning they may not be blood-related but they are as intimate or more at times. This is certainly not unique to gay life, but an interesting form of connection that may have some basis in being an outcast from many—but at the same time, embraced by those who have loving and supportive families of origin.

Kate and I have the relationship of a very close brother and sister, and eventually we I did live together. We both lived in a tenement house where I was upstairs, and she was in the ground-floor apartment. We were the only tenants, and freely moved from apartment to apartment, spending most of our free time together. My career life had found some stability as well with a job as a certified nursing assistant. I had worked as a cosmetologist, in retail, as a courier for a law firm, even as a letter carrier before I found some purpose and passion in healthcare.

Perhaps we all want to give back in an area we are most affected by, or perhaps it was simply a happy accident. I loved my job beyond words, and I was good at it. Kate was a nurse at the same hospital, and we worked graveyard shift together. So, it is not a far stretch of the imagination to see why we formed such a close bond, living and working together—and we bring out the best in one another. We laugh, cry, support, and cherish one another. It is hard for many people to understand how one can be so connected to another person without any romantic connections, but intimacy expressed between best friends is as valuable as intimacy that includes physical or romantic connections. There are many different forms and expressions of love, and these different expressions can be seen working in all areas of life.

Chapter 4

Encountering Abusive Men in the Gay Lifestyle

The sexual and romantic relationships I had with men would quickly become very serious, but always tended to flame out within a matter of weeks or months. Most of these relationships would be abusive in some way. Chris was one of these men, and was in my life when I was living with Kate. He showered me with gifts in the beginning. He bought me a new bedroom set because I had told him how I had so wanted a bedroom to use as a refuge. He also bought me clothes and various pieces of jewelry. He lulled me into a false sense of security with his gifts. Perhaps he sought me out because he was a predator, obsessed with control. Or, perhaps I sought him out because I still had a sense that by *feeling owned and dominated, it made me an acceptable person.*

It doesn't matter what the reason was, because either way, the end result was still the same. I was seeking validation and acceptance from outside sources, rather than from within.

My car's transmission died as I was returning home in the middle of the night from my latest sexual hookup. When Chris found out about it, I lied and said I had been out visiting a friend in crisis. I often used this excuse because in some way it made me feel the way I was trying to prove to the rest of the world I was, placing more value on a perception of self then on the value of being true to oneself. He knew where I had been, he must have. So, the next day, he found a way to step up his ownership of me. He took me to a local car dealership and bought me outright, an almost-brand-new car. He had papers drawn up for me to sign, stating I would pay him back a certain amount every month for five years. I gladly signed. Checkmate!

Less than a week had passed before he became possessive to the point of stalking. He wanted me to account for every minute of my day. He became forceful and violent sexually, and flaunted that if I did not do what he wanted when he wanted, he would make sure the legal ramifications of my signing his promissory note would be swift and severe. Once he told me that I had no idea how much damage he could do to me with all of his "connections." By this time I had begun work with my second therapist, a gay man. I was learning my sexuality was not deviant, or unnatural. The value system of my youth was based on Catholicism, which at its core doctrine demonizes homosexual relationships. I had to let go of those beliefs if I was ever going to fully accept my sexuality as a beautiful and priceless gift, rooted in the very building blocks of life, my DNA.

> **I had to learn I could find value, and in fact God himself in the creation that was me, and the perspective I choose to take of the world around me.**

My new therapist was helping me to find *my own truth,* but change this deep does not happen overnight, and I was still in the throws of being with abusive people. So when this abuse started with Chris, I turned to Kate. I told her what was going on with Chris—all about the emotional and physical abuse, and the sexual abuse and the blackmail. She cried with me, held me so that my fragile state would not derail. The next day a letter from Kate was waiting. It explained she had the means to help, and it was what she wanted to do. Included was a check to get this abusive man out of my life. Kate placed three expectations on the money: 1) I could pay her back only when I was in a financially capable place to do so. 2) I was not to feel indebted to her. She had decided helping me was more valuable than any amount of money, and she had the money to give. 3) Tell Chris to go to hell, and never contact me again. I fulfilled all three demands.

I had felt loved before, but this was perhaps the first time I had ever felt wholly and completely accepted.

Nobody loves you like your mother, and I have a tremendous mother. Family and friends were ample in my life, and they all seemed to love me. Love and acceptance are often bulked together as the same thing, but in my experience, they are not. We can have both, but we put so much stock in our belief systems and our value systems as ultimate truths that we often miss out on the lessons we can learn and experiences we can have by being unwilling to accept certain things about someone, even though we may love them.

The point is: Kate was the first friend I ever had, who, because of the level at which she knew me, fully accepted me…the attributes, the shortcomings, and even the stuff she had no real understanding of on a personal level. She decided I was her brother, and I did not deserve being abused—and that act of love and friendship would prove life saving in the long run. At the time, I was not able to understand it the way I do today. I accepted her generosity, but still it did not change my continual need to be abused and hurt by the men in my life. Regardless, Kate remained my ardent supporter.

A bathhouse is a place where men gather to have sex with other men in one specific place—and I was there often. The bathhouse was set up like a maze of sorts. Corridors were lined with small rooms that included a mattress. It also had a steam room, shower room and some more expensive suites. The lighting is kept to almost nothing and men prowl around in towels, making connections with other men and cruising for sex. Usually anywhere from ten to fifty men were cruising at a time, and it was not a prerequisite to identify outside the bathhouse as gay.

If you had any idea of the number of men who seek anonymous sex with other men while married to, or in a relationship with a woman, you would be truly stunned. I don't believe there is anything intrinsically wrong with casual sex, open relationships, or the various forms of sex play, but the dishonesty of sneaking around while committed to someone else is something I have grown to abhor. It is more pitiable still that those men at the baths who wore wedding bands were dishonest not just with infidelity, but were also living a lie.

But I was myself shackled by shame, and at the time I had no concrete value system of my own. I engaged in sex with anyone who deemed me a worthy sexual partner. This behavior began to falsely validate my worth based on the sexual encounters I had. What obscured my value and belief system at the time was a repression designed to protect myself from the opinions and actions of others, but which lead to dishonesty, and the destabilization of my own sense of self. I have always had great strength in my convictions, but at this time in my life, *I had no convictions, and no real honesty.*

All I had was an unquenchable thirst to be validated and accepted, and the pain of a mental illness that I did not understand beyond public stigma and personal ignorance. Externally, I was kind and caring, giving all I could, and trying to please everyone in the world around me. Inside, I had become enraged, narcissistic, demoralized, and bitter. Resentments were works of art in my mid-twenties, and I was the portrait of an artist I did not even know. Sexually, I was seeking to be submissive for the sake of punishment and lack of control. It was the only drink I could find in those days for my parched, deserted soul. The worst abuse was about to happen. It was a Saturday afternoon when I got a drink my glass simply could not hold—rape.

Was your first thought the same as mine? How does a six-foot-tall, 230-pound man, who is actively seeking to be a submissive sexual object, claim to be raped by another man? It happened, nonetheless, when I was targeted by a predator at that same bathhouse. Both heterosexual and homosexual behavior plays with the roles of dominant and submissive. This can be a beautiful expression of human connection and love, and I don't want anyone to confuse what I am talking about as that. BDSM—includes bondage and discipline (B and D), dominance and submission (D and S), and sadism & masochism (S&M)—is often demonized because it is misunderstood.

Often people don't seem to take the time to learn about things before they place judgment on them. Like in all things, knowledge is power. In this situation however, someone took my choices away. It is never okay to proceed sexually with someone who says "no" for any reason.

I was attacked. I had said, "No!" The man who raped me did so with intent, and he placed a rag of some chloroform substance over my face, just enough to keep me quiet without becoming unconscious. His penis was pierced with a large Prince Albert ring, and with each violent thrust, he ripped my flesh from within. When he was finished, he had the nerve to thank me. There I laid, in a pool of my own blood and his semen, half drugged and in total shock. After some time, I managed to pull myself together and get to my car. Tears would have been salvation, but alas, the ducts were dry. Whatever the pain, I decided it was my fault, and I had to do something, anything to turn my mental attentions elsewhere.

I was scheduled to work that night, and after cleaning myself up at home, Kate and I went in to work together. The ride was silent. She knew I was not okay, but I was not yet willing to talk. I was bleeding internally and barely made it through the shift. When our shift was over and we were back in the car, I could not hold it any longer, and the dam broke. The tears were the most violent I have ever experienced. I was some shadowy version of the self I might have once been, something I had never seen before. The shame did not subside with the tears; it only intensified. We went to the doctor, and I refused to report my circumstance as a rape. I was already humiliated enough having a female doctor examine me anally to document the wounds. She gave me antibiotics, antidepressants, and urged me to seek professional help. I filled the prescriptions, told Kate about what had happened, and retreated to my bedroom—my place of serenity, now filled with the furniture of a prostitute who cared so little for himself he allowed himself to buy into all the bullshit stereotypes he knew, instead of seeking quality professional help—and personal acceptance.

Chapter 5

Detours on the Road to Marrying Mason

One the most important things to realize about therapy is that *it is a process*. This is a much easier concept to wrap one's head around, in a physical sense. Imagine you had an accident, and needed surgery to repair a broken leg. First you would get help for the break. The doctor would set the leg and put a cast on it. For several weeks you would adjust to life on crutches, and you would develop a new routine. The way you bathed yourself, how you got to work, how you prepared your meals, what you did for hobbies—all of this might change while you were dealing with a restricted mobility. Finally the cast would come off, and although the bone might be healed, the leg would be weak from the lack of use of your muscles and tendons, etc. You might go to a physical therapist a couple of times a week to learn exercises to help you rebuild your strength, and you navigate on a leg that had been through a great trauma. It would be a process, and would require you to let go of the old ways of going through your day, without thinking about how you are walking. Suddenly, your consciousness would include paying attention to the obstacles around you, and how you walk.

    The psychological process of therapy is not very different. To move forward, you have to grieve, giving up the old habits of the past, and accept that things are more difficult in the moment. Eventually the way you encounter the world psychologically will become easier. It is not enough to simply act and react without thinking. You have to put more thought into how you live, act, and speak. At the same time, life is still happening all around you. You have no plaster cast to protect you while you heal. So, as you get more and more in touch with who you truly are, and how you want to live your life, you have to, at the same time, try the new ways of acting and reacting, even though you may still be broken, fragile, and not quite healed yet.

Thus, the process is one that does not only affect you, but also all the other people who are in your life. Change starts happening to you and to all around you. I was already engaging in this process during my early to mid-twenties, but I had not yet grasped the idea that my old habitual way of acting and reacting had to change if I was going to heal. My old habits and crutches were still very much in place in my daily life. I did not know this statement would be a mantra about to enter my life in a whole new way. In the fellowships of 12-step recovery rooms, "making the same decisions while expecting different results" is referred to as insanity.

I was coping with trauma by making the same decisions— and expecting different results.

My insanity skyrocketed on a very unexpected afternoon in September of 2006. I was finishing a twelve-hour shift at the hospital. My life had changed drastically from a year earlier when I was raped. I had managed to push most of the trauma from the rape, as well as the years of abusive boyfriends, into a Pandora's box at the bottom of my subconscious. This came at a tremendous cost. I became much more selfish in my daily life, and traded in the support of friends and family like Kate for new man after new man.

The difference was that I had stopped seeking out violent and abusive assholes and instead was looking for "the one." I figured if I could normalize my life to match my adult relationships to the ones I remembered seeing as I grew up that I would find the acceptance I craved. At this time I had found someone who was gentle and sweet. I will call him Mason. He was not very emotional about anything. In the two-and-a-half years we were together, I never saw him cry. I thought I was looking for that kind of guy. Instead of a relationship with someone who I could share my emotions with, I pushed emotions away and found a sweet soul who had very little interest in emotion, at least outwardly.

Kate and I had both moved; I was living with my new boyfriend, now fiancé, after only a month of dating. Kate and I still hung out and saw one another at work, but I soon switched my hours to be on opposite shifts because having this devoted friend and sister around was just too dangerous. I needed everything to appear perfect on the outside, and the only way to do so, was to convince myself inwardly that everything was fine. So instead of conforming as much as I possibly could to what I thought the world wanted of me, in order to be deemed normal. Being normal meant abandoning the deep emotions that had time and time again put people off about me.

My fiancé, whom I married nine months later in an extravagant, over-the-top ceremony in June of 2007, was transgendered. At the time I did not even realize what I was doing. But in retrospect, he was the perfect possible solution. All my years of therapy to this point had helped me change in some very positive ways. I was not willing to suppress my sexuality any longer. I was gay, out, and outwardly proud, and this genie was not going back into any bottle, or closet, in my case. However, subconsciously, I think when I met a man who had been born a woman, it seemed like my best shot at getting total acceptance. Anyone who looked at us knew we were a gay couple, as we were. But somewhere deep inside of me, where the master manipulator lived, I think I believed since my partner was a woman at birth, it made my sexuality acceptable in a way so it did not challenge the old values of my upbringing, while accommodating the new values of my life experience.

I will always be sorry for this. What I did was use this person for my own attempt at finding acceptance, which was a form of abuse in its own way. I have made amends for this by trying to educate others about the immense bravery of the transgendered community. Consciously, I thought I was in love with this man, and in many ways I was. However, if I didn't love myself, *how could I love someone else?* Poorly, that's how.

Anyway, at the very end of that shift in late September, I received a call from another area hospital summoning me there immediately. My maternal grandmother was in the emergency room with chest pains, and the other members of my immediate family were all in Boston helping out with another sick relative. After seeing my grandmother, and speaking with the doctors, I told the rest of the family to stay in Boston. It seemed this was a minor heart episode, and it would result in no more than a night of observation.

The family agreed, and a few hours later I stepped away from my grandmother and into the waiting room of the cardiac care unit, while they settled her in her room for the night. Moments later, the alarms sounded and I heard those all-too-familiar words come over the P.A. system. *Code blue—Code blue.*

I was faced with a decision I was not ready to make. The doctor told me my grandmother had gone into cardiac arrest. Her heart had stopped, and she was not breathing. I needed to make an instant decision about whether I wanted them to use heroic measures to revive her. In shock, and with waves of nausea taking over my body, I had moments to make this life-and-death decision for a woman I dearly loved. It had been five years since my grandfather had passed on, and it seemed she became lonelier and lonelier with every passing day. She was seventy-eight-years old, and her overall health was beginning to decline. I decided to let nature take her to whatever realm was next, and hopefully bring her some peace.

The next week was filled with all the usual demands of burying a loved one. I don't think it was until after we returned home from the burial itself that the trauma of the decision I had made set in. When it did, I was in no way prepared. I had been off all medication for my bipolar disorder for a few years. My abilities had been keenly developed in order to hide the rapid cycling behind my normally high-energy personality, I had earned the trust of all who knew me. I was enrolled in a nursing program, and seemed outwardly to be in a place of relative stability. I would do anything to protect this overall lie, but it was no match for the shame and guilt newly awakened in me, thinking I had made the wrong decision about my grandmother, fearing I had killed her.

Everyone in my family thought I had made the right decision. In fact, she had listed me as someone who could legally make that decision, but that didn't matter. When you awaken shame that's buried in someone, the consequences can be fiercely brutal without the proper support in place. Within a month I was turning to alcohol to soothe the pain of my troubled mind. It was a quick fix, but as alcohol is a depressant, it was not doing a very good job at subduing the feelings I was trying to avoid.

I had pushed away all my friendships in an attempt to keep others from discovering my real pain. My fiancé was working twelve-to-sixteen hour days, often staying in Boston rather than driving back home during the week. I had a lot of time on my hands, my focus on my studies was slowly declining, along with my job performance, and I was becoming more of a regular in the downtown bar scene. I found myself a solution at a particularly sketchy bar. The place was as dirty and unkempt as the clientele. After four hours on the stool, and numerous drinks on my tab, I was freely talking about wanting to do something crazy. When I went into the men's room, a man followed me and offered me my first hit of crack-cocaine. It took less than a second for total feeling of elation and peace, the likes of which I had never known, to wash over me like a typhoon. I was instantaneously transported to a place I had been searching for since the earliest onset of my bipolar symptoms at the age of ten.

In fact, looking back, I realize the sense of relief was even more primal, something I had not felt since before I knew that I was different than most other kids in some ways. It was a feeling predating my father's birds-and-bees talk, when my nine-year-old self realized that I did not have a place in his story. It was a feeling of peace I had not known since before I knew I was gay.

Addiction to Cocaine

Crack is a purer form of cocaine. It is heated in a way to bring the oils of the cocaine into a hardened form. It is then smoked through a small glass pipe, which uses copper mesh as a filter. These "crack pipes" cost only a few dollars, and are sold at convenience stores everywhere. They look like little glass tubes with a flower inside. The copper mesh is a piece of a copper scouring pad. Because of cocaine's purity in crack form, and the more receptive delivery system of smoking as opposed to snorting, the high from crack cocaine is nothing like the high from snorting powder cocaine. The drug enters the body through the lung inhalation, and is then absorbed into the bloodstream. Dopamine, the mood chemical the brain releases during pleasurable experiences such as eating or having sex, floods the mind in a torrent of pleasure. Normally this chemical is reabsorbed by the neurons in the brain that released it. However, the crack inhibits this reabsorption, leaving the brain stimulated by the dopamine. This causes a first-time high you will not reach again—however, the user will never forget it, and will always seek it, no matter what the cost. Even though that first height of pleasure is never achieved again, the drug still creates euphoric highs. The memory of that feeling is what you want to find at any cost. Imagine the best feeling you have ever felt, magnify it by one thousand, and then try to never seek that feeling again. Good luck!

My addiction to this illicit drug was swift, and it caused me immediate damage. I began a life of two faces: in one trying to conceal and hide the torment of my secrets; in the other I fell faster and faster into peril. Both lives were fueled by huge reserves of crack. I managed to conceal my addiction for eight months. Although some people knew something was amiss, they never imagined it was a drug addiction. I was spending hundreds of dollars a week on my drug. I would borrow, beg, and steal for the needed money.

This unchecked addiction was about to collide head on with my wedding to Mason, and be unveiled at last. The week of my June wedding to Mason arrived. I had blown the budget of $20,000 and reached over $40,000, for this three-hundred-guest wedding. All the stops were pulled out, and I spared no cost, no invite. If I could get someone there, I was going to. I believed this way I would feel accepted. Wrong again. The wedding actually consisted of two separate events. One Monday morning in a private ceremony on a beach in Cape Cod, Massachusetts, we legally took our vows in front of a justice of the peace. The party would come later in the week.

Two days later, my addiction was finally revealed when Mason discovered that I was using the internet to connect with other people having sex and using drugs. One of the reasons crack cocaine is called a party drug is because it affects the same area of the brain as the sexual reward center. This part of the brain, called the limbic system, becomes like an intertwined branch. The drug use often becomes synonymous with sex. Inhibitions are lowered to a point where sexual morality of any kind becomes pointless, and boundaries simply don't exist. The brain needs more and more of the drug and the sex to get the same desired feelings of the high. It's a race you can never win, but its participants will run until their body deteriorates to a point of total exhaustion or death. If you are lucky, you will hit bottom, or a place where things are so bad you decide to seek help. It is not hopeless; there is help. However, the vast majority of people are never able or willing to get the help they need, or before they get help, they ruin their lives to such a point of no return that they simply give up.

I had absolutely no clue that I would become a drug addict. In fact, I thought addiction was a disease of poverty, or bad morals. People who were "intrinsically bad" or stupid became drug addicts. You may find yourself reading this and thinking, "I could never be a drug addict, how could someone be stupid enough to let it happen?" Smart people, successful people, professionals from every field of work, and members of every class of life, all struggle with drug addiction. Alcohol is a drug. Smoking is a drug. Food and sex are drugs. Laughter can be a drug, as can drama and hobbies.

Perhaps the most relatable example is the smartphone, which is designed to keep us addicted, always connected and validated. It eases our anxiety to check the screen, and it increases our anxiety when we are away from it.

Everything the human body thinks or does causes a chain reaction of neurological activity in the brain and causes fluctuations in our chemistry. And addiction is chemical dependence. It comes down to simple science: if you are alive, you can become addicted. Some people may have a predisposition, *but that is not a prerequisite.*

People who think that their community is "drug-free" are working within a serious misconception. Every community in every part of the world is susceptible. It was no harder to find and use drugs than it was to go to the grocery store. I smoked it inside and outside. Sometimes it was in palatial homes on wealthy streets, and other times it was in rundown tenement buildings in the poorest sections. I smoked crack while driving, and I smoked crack while working.

This trait was not unique to me. The war on drugs we've heard about is not actually a war on drugs at all, but the overall denial of a culture to treat the underlying problems leading people to moments of great desperation. The weapons we are using in this war are ineffective because they are not treating the underlying causes of the problem. The institutions where most people struggling with chemical dependency can get help are prisons and rehab facilities. In prison there is no real treatment, and in most rehabs, the treatment is not effective as many of clients leave, only to relapse.

Of course that is great for business, and *rehab is a business.* Take a moment to envision a drug addict. We all create a vision based on our own exposure. If you have not been directly impacted or had individual experience with addiction, it may be that your presumptions create a different picture than what is actually there. There is always something psychological and biological going on in the mind and body of a drug addict. Drug use is a behavior and an addiction, both causing crime and killing people. Treating the "drugs" is like bandaging a wound infected with flesh-eating bacteria. If we treat the underlying causes of people choosing to use drugs, along with updated techniques for overcoming addiction, there is a chance the tides will turn in a positive direction.

The night my addiction to crack was uncovered, a devastated Mason wondered how he could have missed the signs, and further wondered if he should go through with this wedding, which had become nothing more than a flaunting of his naiveté in front of everyone he knew and loved. I will never understand why he chose to go forward with it, but he did. He was a victim of my addiction, and he loved me, so he wanted to save me.

Nobody can save an addict who is active in his addiction. The addicted person needs to want to change, and also needs to be fortunate enough to have access to available help.

Even then, there are no guarantees, and many addicts will lose their life, one way or another, to their addiction. Blame at this stage is useless, but our society seems focused on justice and revenge, and the stigma that overcomes the person who seeks help is often as deadly as the drugs themselves. For many, extreme prison sentences for possession eliminate any hope that was left.

Chapter 6

My Husband Insists I Enter Treatment

The wedding went forward, followed by what must have been one of the worst honeymoons in history. Eight days later we were back home to deal with the wreckage. Mason decided if I wanted to make this relationship work, I'd have to meet some demands. They included: I start attending 12-step meetings, get and work with a sponsor, and we go together see a therapist of his choosing. I was to then continue seeing this therapist, but Mason would come only when he felt like he had anything to work on. It was a courageous and generous plan, but it was doomed from the start.

My first meeting was one of Alcoholics Anonymous. I was told at the beginning of the meeting when I was greeted that because I was an addict and not an alcoholic, I was not to speak at the meeting, only listen. This immediately puzzled me, seeing as they professed alcohol to be a drug at the meeting. I was matched up with a sponsor, and we began meeting weekly to read the *Big Book*, a text written in the 1930s by a group of alcoholic men. I had to fill out forms corresponding with the steps as written.

I managed to not use no more than ten days at a time, and when I had relapsed for the third time, my sponsor told me I was not serious about recovery, and he fired me, meaning he would no longer meet with or try to help me. I would not say that every 12-step meeting or sponsor is the same, but I will criticize the damage that can be caused by some of the psychologically unsound parts of using a system of recovery that has not been updated since its original founding, in a different time and place. The only thing standing in the way of change is usually an unwillingness to adapt to change.

Once I was able to figure out that the slogan, "Stick with the winners," was not one I believed in, I was able to hear the other slogans like, "Take what you need and leave the rest." Both are examples of wisdom from the same program, but until I was able to find the strength to use what I needed, I was in trouble. I was also consumed with fear and feelings I did not know how to process, so my vulnerability was both a blessing and a curse.

The new therapist was a woman with whom I not only had a bad connection, but did not particularly like. Our couple's session consisted of me listening to all the ways in which I had destroyed Mason's life, and how the trust that had once been present in our relationship could never be recovered. Life would always be lived under a cloud of suspicion. Understandable. Yes. The only way? No.

Mason decided that he was only responsible to be part of the first session, and after that, the problem was mine to fix. The individual sessions were akin to having a root canal. This therapist would speak to me with her fancy psychological terms, and I would resist her every move at gaining my most intimate thoughts. We were oil and water.

This experience in therapy was a colossal failure. It not only did not make things any better, it cemented the emotional distance between Mason and me. We did the best we could with the cards we were playing, but after seven months of marriage, and many failed attempts at abstinence from crack, it was time to throw in the towel. Mason was despondent with the entire situation, and threw himself into his work. His family wanted him free from me from the start, and he had finally come to the same conclusion. Although I disagreed at the time, it was the best thing that could have happened to either one of us.

I had last used crack cocaine on January 5. After not calling into work, and not showing up for two days, Kate had come to our condo and found the place a mess. Mason was never very interested in anything when he was home except for his own research and writing, so the household chores all fell on me, and I had stopped doing any of them. Filth filled every room, and money and drug paraphernalia were strewn all over the place. I had cashed my paycheck, and in haste took five hundred dollars straight to my dealer. I always bought my drugs this way. I knew eventually I would spend every cent I had on the drugs, but by purchasing it incrementally, this made me feel like I had more control over my use than I did.

Kate managed to come in while I was out making the buy. I will never forget coming back home after the buy. I just knew she had been there, even though she did not disturb anything, and even if she had, I would not have noticed. Sometimes we stumble on moments of intuition in our lives, and this was one of those moments. For a day and a half, I had been dodging phone calls from her and everyone else who cared about me. I knew she would come, but she would not intervene for she knew there was nothing more anyone could do. She saw I was not there, called my then-husband and parents to let them know I was obviously out using, and went home to be alone with her own worry, fear, and anger.

Mason felt obligated to get me to inpatient treatment, so on January 11 he flew with me to Minneapolis, Minnesota. The day before I left I had to replace my license, which I had lost when someone I had used drugs with stole my wallet. My mother had to meet me at the Department of Motor Vehicles with a copy of my birth certificate so I could obtain the new license, and I'd then fly out early the next morning. I will never forget the look on her face as we parted ways. She hugged me goodbye. Her face was red with sadness, and her heart was broken with desperation at the sight of her son who she was terrified she may never see again. The grief was palpable in the cool winter air. I was unshaven, dirty, unmotivated, and had given up on life. Neither of us spoke of it, but I think we both felt this was possibly goodbye for the last time.

Heading to Minnesota for Treatment

In the very early morning hours of January 11, 2008, I began the most unplanned journey of my life. I had chosen to travel to Minneapolis, Minnesota, where I would enter a drug rehabilitation center focused on treating people who were LGBT, and who also struggled with chemical dependency. Mason had given me the new ultimatum to either move out or go into inpatient treatment, and I chose the latter.

The destination was very deliberate. I was so full of shame as a "chronic relapser" I wanted to get as far from my home area as I could. In researching facilities that were both covered by my medical insurance, and appropriate for the hodgepodge of challenges I seemed to be facing, this particular treatment center seemed like it might be the best option.

The day started extremely early. I was to take a cab to the rail station, and take the train to Boston's Logan Airport. I had to be in Boston by four-thirty to get through security and meet up with Mason. He stayed at his parent's house near the airport after work the night before. I staggered out into the snow, exhausted from both desperation and several days without any real sleep. Alas, a week had passed since my last crack use, I was officially on a medical leave of absence from my job. Here I was with Mason again, sitting on the floor of a terminal in the airport, awaiting a flight to Minneapolis. The land of ten thousand lakes is often referred to in the 12-step rooms as the land of ten thousand treatment centers. It seems Minnesota has more drug treatment options per capita than most states.

Mason and I parted ways almost immediately after arriving at the treatment facility. He could not seem to get away from me fast enough. I was a tornado of drama. If I wasn't apologizing for my almost unforgivable behaviors while using, I was bawling and begging him not to leave me, or worse still, firing all of my rage and confusion over this addiction in bouts of venomous verbiage.

Very frequently, persons in the throws of chemical use are fueled by incredible shame and humiliation. While actively using our drug or drugs of choice, we deflect all of the responsibility for our use. This is not just because we are selfish assholes, as is often appears. If I admitted to myself the reality of my behaviors before I was ready to do so—I had been an adulterer, a thief, a liar, a drug addict in the throws of his addiction—I think I would have been left with zero will to live.

Creating a false reality, whether consciously or subconsciously, about what is really happening, and deflecting ownership of our own behavior, is often a survival technique.

Sometimes we have to accept the truth of a situation a little bit at a time so we are not consumed by it. In the case of drug users, *something drastic has to happen* to make them fully aware of what their addiction is doing to them and to the world around them. Sometimes this happens due to an intervention, and sometimes it happens when an event or series of events happen that are so bad it causes the addict to take a cold, hard look at what his use and its surrounding behaviors is causing. This can be anything from contracting an illness, overdosing, or losing things or people.

Many addicts and former addicts refer to this as hitting their "rock bottom." Getting help for chemical addiction is not like getting help for many other ailments. No pill exists to make it better, and usually compassion for the person who is suffering is mixed with feelings of anger over the behavior itself. We have usually burned most of our bridges by the time we seek the help, and what we have available for help is not very good. Some people are able to stop using, and never go back, but they are in the great minority. Most will find that the journey to a life of not abusing chemicals is often as tumultuous as the trauma of using.

Many different avenues of seeking help are available—from stopping cold turkey to 12-step recovery programs, counseling, even some medicinal aids to transition to not using substances abusively, or harm reduction. However, the underlying truth is that the person himself needs to find something more important than the drugs and their effects to hold onto in order to make the necessary changes in his choices and behaviors. It is never as simple as just stopping. I was not aware when Mason dropped me off that it was the last gasp of breath left in my marriage to him. He turned me over to the professionals at the treatment center in Minnesota, and he flew out the same afternoon to carry on with his life, and try to make sense of the last year with me.

Chapter 7

My Treatment Program and Sober-House Living

Inpatient treatment meant a rigorous schedule of meetings and groups, assessments and journaling. The model used in this facility at the time was based on a 12-step program. This model is a list of twelve step-by-step instructions for the person who wants to use abstinence as the perfect model of sobriety. It is one of some success.

In the 1930s, two alcoholics put together this program in order to stay sober, and it has spread across the globe, but has changed very little over the years. These men were not professionals in the field of chemical dependence, but rather a group of addicts and egoists whose open value system was based in the belief that there is a God, *and they were not God.* They could never stay sober on their own, and had to continuously share their experiences with alcohol and life with one another and others who struggled with alcoholic drinking.

A main tenet of their program for sobriety was being of service to one another, and to humanity in general. If they could find a way to turn their worries over to a god of their own understanding, while contributing to society in service of others, and sharing their humanity with one another, they had a good chance of being able to resist taking the first drink. That drink opened their Pandora's box, or as they referred to it, aggravated their "allergy" to alcohol. The allergy is a compulsion to keep drinking, one so strong it usually took them to the darkest corners of their psyche and the world. By talking with one another every day about their personal resentments toward others and the world around them, they could find some serenity with life, and also find a greater meaning in not drinking than they did in drinking. By having a spiritual life, they could give up some of their need to always be in control of everything around them, changing the focus from being entirely on the "self," and instead reaching out to others in the greater world.

Their fellowship grew and spread and today, as a worldwide organization, it still attracts innumerable people who attend countless meetings a year. Most countries and most subcultures have their own meetings, based on the steps and traditions the original two men developed, and many people are able to use this system as a guideline to get their lives back from the horrors of addictive drinking and drug using.

I was a big supporter of the 12-step model, and in fact I attended meetings at least once a day. I have "worked the steps," and I have been sponsored and been a sponsor. I am not, however, a believer that the way one person uses this program is the *only or best way* to overcome or manage his chemical dependence issues.

After several successful years of being an active participant in the 12-step model, I found that it was no longer working for me, and that while much of what I gained from participation in this program was positive, it was no longer something I could accept *without question*. So instead I became a member of the "harm-reduction" method. I will go into this in greater depth later.

I think there are as many ways to overcome active addiction, as there are people addicted to something. The wisdom of time has shown me that being open minded to all ideas is most helpful. Try different ways to live your healthiest life, and if they don't work for you, put them gently aside, with the respect they deserve. What works for me may not work for you, and vise versa. The meetings can be a great way to share these different strategies and ideas, but too often people find themselves all caught up in perfectly working what is referred to as "the program," and once again the wisdom gets traded in for an unhealthy ego. I did this many times myself. I would try so hard to work a perfect program, and when I made minor mistakes, these issues would inflate to a size I could not handle. To me it meant I was not working a good program, and I was again, in my consciousness, a colossal failure. But, even failure can bring self-validation.

Some people never encounter this problem, and for them, 12-step recovery remains an invaluable tool. The reason I said failure can bring self-validation is because it genuinely does. So many times we resort to methods of behavior that is detrimental to ourselves as a species, or on a personal level, because we know these behaviors. Actions however, speak a language so much stronger than actual words.

I have never heard anyone say: give me more pain, more trials, and struggles to cope with in my life.

What I mean by this is best expressed in this little anecdote. Take a moment to think about someone in your life who seems to have the worst luck of anyone you know. Maybe it is a friend, a relative, or a co-worker. Who it is doesn't matter, but think about this certain person you know who often seems to be a victim. Time after time you might ask this person a simple question like, "How are you doing?" and you get a response filled with the ways in which the world is treating him badly. His paycheck was late, and all his bill payments bounced. He has another physical ailment to contend with even though he recently got over the flu. Every time he goes into the city, he get a parking ticket. His doctor is incompetent, or no matter how hard he tries to diet, he never seems to lose an ounce of weight. In fact, while on this latest diet he gained five pounds after having an allergic reaction to some new food on the new diet plan.

We all know someone like this. Some people are drawn to this type of personality, while others are repelled by it. Likely everyone you know who knows this person would probably agree he is the unluckiest person alive. I used to feel that way, and in fact it led to the deepest moments of desperation I have ever known. This is exactly how I felt when I arrived in Minnesota for inpatient chemical dependency treatment. I was a beaten man, trying to understand how a person who meant so well, as I always did, had ended up in this hell. At the time I did not understand I simply had created the life I was living, and I was getting enough validation from those around me for my hardships so I was no longer even trying to create a happier life for myself. I was surviving, not succeeding, and only barely surviving at that.

We all need to have a purpose if we want to keep going. The purpose I had come to rely on was one of being a failure; therefore, a chronic relapser, a sick man who chose self-punishment over self-reliance. I had a purpose… I had never come to fully understand my bipolar disorder; therefore I could never begin to learn how to live with it, instead of living against or in spite of it. I had yet to truly understand the grace in being a human expression of a beautiful spirit. I chose instead to buy into a well-meaning, but fear-based faith that said I was not gay, but rather I was a sinner. Therefore, every time I would make some very uphill progress at deciding to make healthy and responsible decisions for myself, I would inevitably realize subconsciously that I truly thought of myself as a sinner, a madman, and a drug addict—and I was good at it. I was good at screwing up everything, bouncing back, and then when things started to turn around, screwing up again.

I created my own reality, and I needed someone professionally trained to help me realize all of this. It would happen in its own time, at its own pace, and with lots of mistakes made along the way.

What was important, and perhaps the reason why my addiction did not kill me, was I had to keep showing up and trying everything I could to truly understand who I really was, what I believed, and why by being alive, *I had purpose.*

It is important to state that I do not want to bring an indictment upon treatment and sober house systems. Rather I feel I need to highlight the challenges of receiving appropriate and accessible healthcare, which often requires intensely proactive work for one's own healthcare needs. A lot of red tape needs to be cut in order to effectively navigate many advantages of these varied healthcare opportunities. I believe in, have experienced, and support 12-step recovery, harm reduction, sober housing, and treatment centers for addictions. However, to understand how I achieved this open-mindedness to and gratitude for all of these available options, it is important to highlight some of the challenges I faced early on, and important to understand not only my story, but the extent of the obstacles in an imperfect system. Sober housing works for some people, and in many ways, it worked for me, but it is neither perfect nor well studied. It is, in my opinion, the best option we sometimes have, but that does mean we *should not try* to find a better way.

Twelve-step treatment and sober-living houses can be and are often very useful tools in communities throughout the world. Some of my greatest psychological progress was made through sharing my experiences in early recovery with others going through the process at the same time, and treatment is often very enlightening. If willpower were enough, most addicts would conquer their addictions with great haste. But willpower alone is never enough to turn away from a learned behavior that brings definite psychological rewards. In the many years that I have been in recovery, I have buried more friends than I can remember. Most of these deaths have been from overdose, suicide, or desperation.

Too many people are still dying from their addictions—and as a society, we should not accept that what we have for treatment and help is working well. I went to inpatient treatment three separate times the first year. I also lived in two different sober houses, as well as trying to do it on my own.

The biggest problem I had, and continue to have with the systems in place to help has to do with 1) the lack of professional help being readily available, and 2) the challenges surrounding being honest. Treatment centers are all over the country. With various systems and programs, my inpatient experience was with the same treatment center all three times. These programs are generally about twenty-eight days long. However, some programs are as short as ten days, and other as long as a couple of years. The longer programs are seldom covered by insurance, so the need for self-funding often prohibits many people from entering a long-term program. In total I have spent four extended periods in treatment centers, once for ten days, twice for twenty-eight days, and once for forty-five days.

The twenty-eight day model I experienced was composed of a rigorous daily schedule of groups and meetings, usually an hour or two in length, and moderated by a chemical dependency counselor. These counselors are, at a minimum, trained in a standard two-year program, and often are very competent. Many are in recovery themselves. However, because addiction is frequently the symptom of underlying mental health challenges, it can be hard for someone not properly trained in psychological or psychiatric care to provide the range of care needed for many patients. In fact, much of the most helpful work in this environment comes from the relationships and sharing between patients themselves.

I did have some access to mental health professionals while inpatient. In fact, I met my current psychiatrist and psychologist while in treatment. They were not on staff, but came in once a week to work with patients at the facility. This is where I met Kathy Vader, my psychologist. But both the relationship with her and with my psychiatrist would have just been twenty-minute assessments had I not had the initiative as well as the financial means to seek out these professionals' services after I left the facility. The likelihood is not high for most newly sober and fresh-out-of-treatment people to have access to, or have had chance introductions with, competent professionals in mental healthcare while in treatment. This is another example of the need for proactive healthcare.

Each time I returned for another inpatient treatment, I did so because *not choosing treatment* would have prohibited me from being able to get back into sober housing, which I saw as my only opportunity to avoid homelessness. I was in no condition to be able to hold a job in those days. My parents were, with great personal sacrifice, in the position to help me, and the best knowledge they or I had at the time was that sober housing was the way to go.

The local treatment centers often have a list of area sober houses they can recommend. The client then makes an appointment to "interview" with one. If the members and manager of the sober house decide that the client is a good risk, and deserves a chance, the client is then offered a spot in the house. There is no real relationship other than the referrals the treatment center and sober houses give back and forth to one another.

Although the treatment facility has some adequate professional care, I found there was none to speak of in the sober house system I experienced. As you will see in the coming case notes, I would be kicked out of a sober house for breaking the rules because I was using, and then I would have to go back into inpatient treatment to be able to resume having a place to live. Advice was available, and there was often assistance to try and get me to the help I needed, but this was not professional advice from qualified mental healthcare workers, and there was no obligation on the part of anyone associated with the house to follow through with my capability to access the help.

Once I moved into a sober house, I needed to put down a deposit equal to one month's rent. This is not a security deposit, but is a "sober deposit." The consequence of using and being honest about it, no matter how brief or extensive the use was or how devoted to trying sobriety again, resulted in forfeiting this sober deposit, and being immediately kicked out of the house. Locks were changed at once, and other residents bagged up my personal belongings in order to open the bed for a new resident. I was not allowed to move back in unless I: 1) returned to and completed a treatment program, 2) was able to come up with another sober deposit, 3) was re-interviewed by the house manager and residents, 4) house residents voted to approve my return, and 5) gained the approval of the owner. This caused me and many other people who struggled with relapse in their early recovery to bounce back and forth, or to lie about having used in order to try and maintain some form of housing.

Of course these rules come not *only* from profit motive, but also provide protection for all residents of the house—for they are often deeply affected by being confronted with someone's active use, while in a state of great vulnerability themselves. However, once again this highlights the need for less of a black-and-white mentality, and more of a spectrum of options for how to handle early recovery struggles, which are as varied as the people experiencing them. Perhaps this fact best demonstrates why sober houses should be required to have an mental health professional on hand for all of its residents. This would allow everyone who is living there to navigate the perils of addiction and relapse in a productive way. It is my opinion, and I think it is one of common sense, that having psychiatrists and psychologists associated with sober housing would allow countless more people to survive and flourish as productive, non-using members of their communities and society.

Sober living has almost no regulations, and it is not working well enough.

Here is what my first year looked like once I arrived in Minnesota on January 2008:

- January 2008: 28-day inpatient treatment for $30,000 (insurance accepted)
- Early February: Discharged to sober house for $600 sober deposit plus $600 first month's rent
- Late February: Relapse; reported it to house: loss of sober deposit, back to treatment: $30,000 (insurance accepted)
- Late March: Discharged; sober house refused to reaccept
- Sober house two: $575 sober deposit plus $575 first month rent plus $25/week for household sundries
- Early May: Relapse; attempted to hide having used, kicked out of house, loss of sober deposit, broke. Began living in car. No longer insured. Prostituted myself for money, infected with HIV. Qualified for state-funded treatment due to HIV status. 30 days inpatient treatment: ($30,000–or whatever state paid)
- Late May: Moved into own apartment: $850 security deposit and $850 first month's rent
- Late October: Hospitalized for systemic infection due to IV-drug use; defaulted on apartment and readmitted to inpatient treatment. Loss of security deposit. Treatment cost: $45,000 for 45-day stay

–November: Discharged from treatment back to sober house one: $600 sober deposit and $600 first month's rent

This is the revolving door where I learned to dance to the system's rules. I am not saying the addict should have no consequences for using when he has entered into a contract not to. I am saying the treatment centers are some of the very things in those early months that were supposed to be the most helpful—but almost became the most deadly.

I was attending seven-to-ten 12-step meetings a week. I was living in a sober house with other newly recovering addicts, and I was adjusting to a life in a new city *where my housing relied on residents' relapse to keep making more money*. Although a license is required, and ordinances are in place to follow in order to own and operate a sober house, no real law states that there needs to be accessible counseling or mental health care available. In my case, there was not, and I was out of money, living with destroyed credit, and officially not on any health insurance policy.

My saving grace turned out to be another chronic disease. Sometime before entering my third treatment program, I found myself homeless for the first time in my life. I was receiving some financial help from my parents, and I worried if I told them I had been kicked out of my sober house for using, they might stop supporting me financially. I had no job, no solid support network yet in Minnesota—and no grip on sanity. Mason had started divorce proceedings back east. I agreed he could have everything, not that we had a whole lot to sort out. I would not contest the divorce in any way, but he would have to pay for the legal fees as I had no means to help. I was living out of my car, my only worldly possession. I would spend the day hopping from coffee shop to AA meeting to coffee shop, until it got to be dark. Then I would hang out in some areas known for drug traffic and prostitution. This is how I survived those few weeks as a homeless person. I would do what I knew how to do well to make money. I had become a prostitute for money and/or drugs. It was not difficult to find guys who wanted to get me high, and use me sexually. All I needed to know was where to look—and what "the look" actually meant. Having a laptop made things easier because I would connect with most of my "sexual clients" on internet sex-hookup sites.

The damage that living as a homeless prostitute caused to my psyche was swift and harsh. I would do anything to get whatever someone would pay, and I was eager to use any drug offered. This is how I was first introduced to crystal meth. I had never used meth before, but while in treatment with meth addicts, I had quite an education about what it would do, and the ways to use it most effectively.

My first time using was intravenously. I still preferred the high of crack cocaine. Most addicts form a biochemical relationship with a certain substance, and it becomes "their drug of choice." Meth did not bring me to the same mental place as crack, but rather to a place where I lost all inhibitions and ability to make sound decisions, other than those that would continue to fuel my insatiable need for more drugs and sex.

Crystal methamphetamine is "cooked." It is made from pseudoephedrine and things like tractor fluid, and is a very crude drug. It is completely toxic, causes people to lose teeth, develop internal injuries, succumb to damage of all organ systems, and the list goes on. The high is not as disgusting as the ingredients. People inject meth into their bloodstream, snort it, smoke it, and even use it rectally. Every method of use elicits a slightly different high. The IV use of meth produces the fastest, most intense, and most damaging high. Its effects impact the entire central nervous system, and a feeling of total euphoria and sexual overdrive occurs instantaneously.

After the high wears off, the brain becomes totally depleted—and inexplicable depths of depression and desperation ensue, sometimes for days or weeks. In many ways, continued use becomes about avoiding this desperation, much the same way heroin use often becomes about not getting physically sick from withdrawal.

Almost immediately I was in a full manic episode—no sleeping, no eating, no caring for anything but staying high at all costs. This is also when the mania part of my bipolar disorder turned fully away from having any positive connotations, and became solely a never-ending energy and desire to self-destruct. Previously, mania had caused me to make irrational decisions and lash out in anger, but also I would be intensely creative during manic episodes. Now it was all about obliterating any healthy or positive thing in my life. It was about knowing the mania would soon end, and the depression would be utterly debilitating. It meant living in a state of suicidal thoughts, but not having the internal drive to abruptly end my life.

I was trying to kill myself with the drugs…but I was not dying. I was on a collision course with a horrifying suicide solution that would permanently change my life in a different way than I thought. While I was surfing the web at an Internet café, I was picked up by a guy online. He had plenty of meth to shoot me up with, and was also offering to pay me forty dollars. All he asked in return was to allow him to shoot me up with the same needle he used on himself, and that I let him tie me up and use me sexually until he decided to ejaculate inside of me. He was HIV-positive, and wanted to infect me. I don't remember exactly what thoughts were going through my head when I decided to go to his apartment and consent to his demands.

In hindsight I can plainly see my willingness to allow this stranger to shoot drugs into me, and infect me with HIV, *was an absolute suicide attempt on my part*—a perfect solution for a shattered mind and quickly dying body. If I died accidentally from overdose, or if he would tie me up and then kill me, or if I left with only forty dollars and a deadly disease, I would achieve the suicide, the idea running like a fantasy show nonstop through my restless mind. I wanted to die, but could not find the ability to do it myself.

Perhaps the truth of the matter is that I was too strong-willed, stubborn, or just plain scared to allow myself to do the deed. Whatever happened, this moment would result in my death, which was all I needed to know and all I really wanted, so I wasted no time. Several years later while still living in Minneapolis, occasionally I'd find myself driving past the building where this experience happened. A sense of sadness still comes over me when I do, but more important, I have a strong sense of self-respect and empowerment. *I would not have made the same choice today, but today I am in a much healthier place.*

Even when I face manic episodes today, I have suicidal thoughts. The difference is that I know it will pass, it always does. It might be very painful, and I may not be able to control the thoughts of killing myself, but I have a sense of purpose, a strong support system, and the benefit of time and experience.

Chapter 8

HIV-positive—and a New Therapist

Human Immunodeficiency Virus (HIV) leads to Acquired Immunodeficiency Syndrome (AIDS). Some thirty plus years after its discovery, a life-altering stigma is still attached to people who are infected. HIV can be contracted by anyone, and is transmitted through the direct exchange of bodily fluids carrying the virus, specifically blood, semen, and vaginal secretions. It is not a bad person's disease, or one contracted exclusively by drug addicts or homosexual men. Women, heterosexuals, professionals, people who have never taken a drink or used a drug; all classes and cultures have people in their ranks who are living and thriving with HIV. This also includes many people who have the virus and are chronically ill, or do not have access to the necessary medical care and support systems.

I have to admit that at first I was not well informed. It had never directly affected me, and I never took the time to really learn anything in depth about HIV or AIDS. Eventually I got educated about the disease, and took charge of my healthcare related to it, but it took many years for me to fully come to terms with being HIV-positive. To this day I still have times where I struggle to accept HIV and its effects on me personally and others who live with it.

It is easy to look at the challenges in life and think that things are unfair, and have happened to us. My truth is: I was born with challenges, which are at times unique, but most of all are part of the human experience. I once heard someone say: "We are not in this life for peace." This is a reality. Being at peace with oneself is attainable, but it takes work and constant self-evaluation. *The good in life is not as good without the bad*—and I have learned more about myself through times of crisis than I could ever dream of while in times of static contentment.

The real solution for me was coming to understand and embrace all of these converging lessons—and turn them into opportunities. I do not do that perfectly by any means, but over time and with great practice, I have come to see my life as an opportunity. How I have done this has been in the form of the therapeutic process, and my work with Kathy Vader greatly helped me process it all. Fortunately, access to the full scope of healthcare that I needed became granted when I became HIV-positive. Because I had no income, was unable to hold down a job at the time, and thus no insurance, I became covered by state-funded programs that would allow me to obtain the healthcare I needed to heal and become the functional, sustainable, and capable self I always hoped I could be. It was going to take a lot of persistence, the desire to be and live in a state of health, and a whole lot of trust in my relationship with this new asset of mine, Kathy Vader, L.P.

NOTE: Any time Kathy's words are used, they are in a different type.

Meet Kathy Vader, L.P.—Daniel's Therapist

As a Licensed Psychologist with a private practice, consisting primarily of LBGT adults, many of my clients also have substance abuse issues. When people ask me how I ended up specializing in this population, I often say, "The Holy Spirit has a sense of humor."

I was a wife and mother for many years, marrying right after graduation from college. After my five children were in school full-time, I started volunteering in the court system, working with both juvenile and adult offenders. In 1979, I became a full-time probation officer, and worked in this capacity for eighteen years. In 1983, I decided I wanted a Masters Degree, and earned an M.A. in Theology from St. Catherine's University in 1986. After another year and a half, still a probation officer, I began a Psychology

Masters program at St. Mary's University, graduated in 1991, and became licensed in 1993.

Early on in my private practice, a friend who is also an LP, asked me to work part-time at Pride Institute, an LGBT, inpatient chemical dependency program. I had known very few gay people up until this time, but immediately became "hooked" on this population. I loved my work at Pride, and eventually became the psychologist there, a position I held for thirteen years. So, I am not gay, not in recovery, and have been a practicing Catholic my whole life.

My theory about working with this population—when I don't share their issues—is that there is no possibility of countertransference. Yes, I have to listen very carefully, and try to understand each person who comes for therapy. I can't rely on, "I know what it's like to be gay, alcoholic, etc." I have to try my best to get inside their heads, to see the world as they see it, without any preconceived ideas. Transference and countertransference are issues that as a psychologist I must continually be aware of.

Transference refers to the redirection of a client's feelings about a significant person to the therapist. This can be sexual, but in my experience, transference most often manifests itself in clients projecting onto me their feelings toward their mothers. I am roughly the age of their mothers (or in some cases…their grandmothers) so this is a pretty natural thing to happen. Transference can actually be a very helpful thing in therapy *if* it is recognized, accepted, and discussed.

One long-standing client lied to me about using meth one time because, as we discussed later, he was so afraid of my disapproval or even worse, abandonment. I explained to him that abandonment was not part of my therapeutic process, and that honesty was crucial to our relationship.

It is not surprising that clients who have had negative experiences when sharing some shameful (in their opinion) behavior would withhold or minimize what they have done. When they test out my offer of being totally honest, with no judgment from me, it may be the first time they have ever experienced this unconditional acceptance.

Countertransference, in a way, is *the opposite of transference in that is the redirection of a therapist's feeling toward her client.* If clients bring up primary relationship issues that are similar to my own, I first acknowledge these feelings and then realize this is a normal occurrence in therapy. My feelings do not have to be shared with the client, but I have to put them aside, and remind myself that my experiences are not necessarily those of the client.

Countertransference can also occur when the therapist has experienced a similar problem as the client has, and over-identifies to the point of saying, "This is what worked for me when I had this issue, so it will probably work with you." I see this occurring with 12-step sponsors at times—they have the shared experience of chemical addiction, and are now experiencing a period of sobriety, which can be very encouraging to the person they sponsor (sponsee). The problem arises when the sponsor supports only one way of getting sober—his way—without understanding that the sponsee may need an alternate approach to his own chemical health.

My theoretical base is Humanistic-Existential. I probably do something different with each client, and I let each one lead the way to what we discuss. Carl Rogers, the American psychologist who is among the founders of the humanistic approach to psychology, used, "unconditional positive regard," which comes pretty naturally to me. I don't try to force change, but provide an atmosphere where change can take place. This approach fits perfectly with using harm reduction when working with clients with chemical issues. Because each client is unique, the path to chemical and emotional health is different for each one.

Why Humanistic-Existential Therapy Methods Benefit My Clients

During my graduate studies in psychology at St. Mary's University, I took a class in Cognitive-Behavior therapy (CBT) concurrently with Humanistic-Existential therapy. I knew nothing about this approach, but the CBT professor was intelligent and a very good teacher. In one of the first classes, he told us that CBT was the way to go, because insurance companies weren't paying for long-term therapy, and therefore we needed a short-term, goal-directed approach. As the class progressed, we were taught the principles of thinking errors (cognitive distortions) and their relationship to feelings and behaviors. The therapeutic process involves the therapist pointing out the client's thinking errors, challenging these beliefs, and helping the client see these beliefs as hypotheses rather than facts. The desired result is that once a client recognizes his thinking errors, he will be motivated to change his behavior. Much of the class was spent doing role-plays with other students, practicing this technique.

NOTE: This in itself is part of the cognitive-behavior process because a client engaged in CBT will be expected to do homework or practice outside of sessions.

From the beginning, I was *very* uncomfortable doing this exercise because I felt in such a deep way it did not fit for me. Because I was so early in the Master's program, and also because it seemed every other student in this class was thrilled with CBT, it was very difficult to share my feelings. I had to figure out a way to do well in the class, and at the same time be honest about the theory not being right for me.

My final paper was entitled, "Cognitive Behavioral Therapy for the Existential Humanist." I don't remember the details, but I focused on how some CBT techniques could be used in specific goal-oriented situations that might arise in therapy. It must have worked because I got an A, and although the professor still thought I was being unrealistic, he praised my creativity.

As I began the class in Humanistic-Existential theory, I knew I had found my niche. Dr. H. was a brilliant teacher with a PhD, who also had a private practice. Dr. H not only taught the humanistic approach, but also lived it in the way she taught. At the end of each class, she would ask for a volunteer to act as a client with whatever real issue she felt comfortable discussing. Dr. H would then proceed to do a magical mini-session. In those few minutes, she would connect with the student with such depth it appeared they had been doing therapy together for years. I knew in every part of my being *this* was how I wanted to practice psychology.

Additionally, I took two classes in Jungian psychology, named after Carl Gustav Jung, a Swiss psychiatrist and psychoanalyst who founded analytical psychology. He came to the attention of Viennese founder of psychoanalysis, Sigmund Freud, and they then collaborated. This teaching could not have been more opposite from the CBT class, and Dr. J, also a private practitioner, was our professor. He was casual about seeing clients "for years," and somehow insurance, or some other means, paid for it. He said you could never do Jungian-depth psychology short term, and he refused to live by arbitrary insurance rules. He evidently made a living doing the type of therapy he loved.

While at St. Mary's, we were urged/required to finish our studies with a strong theoretical base. Being "eclectic" was not acceptable. With a humanistic-existential theoretical base, I can use other techniques, as the situation requires. As an example, I often use basic Relapse Prevention techniques that are cognitively based. Occasionally, a new client will ask me what type of therapy I "do." I love this question, but feel at a loss to accurately describe what I do actually "do."

Humanistic Therapy assumes the patient has the internal resources to improve, and is in the best position to resolve his/her dysfunction. This therapy is truly "client-centered," which means I do something different with each person. My goal is to understand this person's view of the world, and consider his/her behavior in this context.

Many clients will ask, "*Why* do I do these things?" I dissuade the client from asking "why," and suggest "how" is a better question. And there *is* a difference. "Why did you do this?" implies blaming, but "How could this happen?" leaves a lot of room for discussion and understanding. I love to quote St. Paul, "Why is it the evil I don't want to do, I do—and the good I want to do, I don't do?"

To make mistakes is totally human, keeps us grounded in our own imperfection, and challenges us to learn from these mistakes, and make better choices in the future. Alcoholic Anonymous (AA) calls these imperfections "character defects," which has seemed unduly negative to me. It is *not* a defect of character to stray from a path of perfection, but a sign of our humanity. How can we experience empathy if we have not embraced our own "shadow side"? Deeply rooted in Jungian psychology is the belief that we all have a "shadow side"—a part of us we would prefer to keep hidden and secret. It is by not only accepting this part of ourselves but embracing it, can we then modify its influence in our lives.

For me, existentialism implies looking for the meaning of things—searching, discovery, exploration, trial and error, struggle, choice, acceptance—not *one* meaning, but a multiplicity of potential meanings in flux. A good example of existentialism is the meaning of sex for couples. I have seen men who have been together for years, but have never discussed what sex means for them. Unfortunately, this comes to light after one of the partners is discovered having sex with other men outside of their relationship. When confronted, the "acting-out" man will say, "Sex with those other guys means nothing. It is only a physical connection, and has nothing to do with OUR relationship." The other partner is then quite stunned, saying, "I assumed we were monogamous because sex to me should only be in the context of our committed relationship."

Just as many straight couples never discuss having children before they marry, it is surprising to me that many gay couples never know what each other's values are regarding sex. Existentialism is all about what it is to be human—to know that life is hard, full of heartbreak, anxiety, and even guilt. The goal is to accept this reality, and deal with it with compassion, commitment, and purpose.

The meaning of pain is at the core of existentialism—with pain comes growth and even new life. As clients become chemically and emotionally healthier, they become intrigued with the question "Why am I here?" By pondering this question, it is then possible to begin creating a purposeful life.

As I stated before, it is difficult to explain the actual process of Humanistic-Existential therapy. Since I work better with examples, here is one: Bobby came for therapy two years ago after being recently diagnosed with HIV. He had also suffered some heart-breaking professional experiences, and when his primary support group turned on him, he said he had become a virtual recluse, and was afraid to be out in public for fear of being humiliated. Bobby came to his first session with his face almost totally covered by his hat, with his coat collar pulled up over his mouth. As he told his story, I had some doubt about the details he described, but accepted whatever the "facts" were that his situation was traumatic for him. Bobby's family of origin was horrifying—his mother left him with his dad when he was a young child, but took his two sisters with her. She refuses to have any contact with Bobby, as does his father, although both are alive, well, and live in Minnesota. Bobby had been seeing another psychologist for several sessions who was not interested in hearing his story, but instead gave written assignments from a workbook.

After becoming frustrated with this procedure, and realizing it was not helpful, he terminated this course of therapy. I gave Bobby credit for knowing what he did and didn't need, and then told him of my two requirements for therapy: 1) people show up, and 2) they talk—and talk he did. Session after session, Bobby would talk, cry, get angry, and tell me more and more about his childhood as well as his current life issues. It was alarming that he had refused HIV medication, although his numbers were not good. He preferred some holistic approaches (vitamin, natural supplements, etc.), and said he didn't fear death since his present life was so miserable.

Although this was a scary thing to hear, for the time being I accepted his decision. As time went on, the first change Bobby made was to walk his roommate's dog outside every day. This was never suggested, but Bobby said, "Maybe I should get out a little more," even though he still feared running into old acquaintances. Also remarkable was how Bobby's appearance changed; he was clean-shaven, and no hat covered his face when he came for appointments.

Then, at the beginning of one session, he said, "I went to the Mall of America, and bought a few new clothes." WOW, that mall is always full of people, plus it required him to take the light rail to get there and back. A few months later, another miracle occurred, when he finally received Social Security disability, he decided to use his first check to go to California.

The trip was not as successful as he had hoped, because the friend he went to visit basically stood him up. Despite this setback, he got a motel room and went to the ocean do some sightseeing on his own. We meet every two weeks, and he continued to talk about his past and current life. Then Bobby changed infectious disease doctors, and when the new doctor suggested medication, he complied. His HIV numbers changed for the better, and while he still continues with some holistic approaches, he is absolutely med-compliant.

The most recent change occurred when Bobby decided to go back to school. He went through all the preliminary steps to obtain financial aid, and is beginning his second semester in a graphic design program. Bobby has earned A's in each class, and his only complaint is that so many students are not taking the work seriously—and he definitely is. His ultimate goal is to be self-sufficient financially, which would allow him his own living space, and maybe even to move from Minnesota.

What's so remarkable: I initiated none of the changes Bobby had made. While I cannot totally explain how this works, I know forcing change doesn't work. I believe by allowing the person the freedom to make his own choices, very often the choices he makes are good ones. Clients will often say something like "I know you'll be proud of me because I haven't used in two weeks." I discourage this as gently as I can, pointing out that my being proud is not the goal, and they don't have to "perform" well in order to be fully accepted. This is a significant issue because many clients have come from homes where parents demanded nothing short of perfection from their children, and in turn the children would work ceaselessly to gain their parents' love.

Working with Daniel—Started May 9, 2008

My journey with Daniel has been challenging, joyful, scary, and enlightening. One thing has been constant throughout: Daniel has never lost contact with me. Whether depths of depression, the heights of mania, or the throes of addiction, he has stayed connected. Many times with Daniel, as with other clients, I have struggled with having the "right" words to say. When it happens, I have to remind myself that my presence and attention is all I have to offer—*and maybe that's enough.*

What I am absolutely convinced: I learn far more from my clients than they do from me. "He has the map of Ireland written all over his face." This very old saying came to my mind when I first met Daniel. At twenty-eight-years old, Daniel was a patient at an inpatient treatment center for chemical dependency. This was our first introduction, but it was brief. I was responsible for assessing the clients at the treatment facility, and assigning them to work therapeutically with my interns while they were in treatment. I worked there only on Wednesdays, as an adjunct addition to my own practice.

My first actual session with Daniel was four months later when he contacted me about my private practice in Edina, Minnesota. Daniel was living in a sober house in Minneapolis, and was struggling with his chemical health, and had just tested HIV-positive. He believed he had *sero-converted* as a result of illicit drug use and unprotected sex, but had a difficult time remembering the details of the previous few months.

Sero-conversion is the time in which a person first develops antibodies for HIV. They will not yet test positive on an HIV test. It means your sero status is in the process of being converted from HIV-negative to HIV-positive. This usually occurs about ten days after infection—about 80 percent of people get symptoms (heavy cold or flu) and 20 percent do not.

Sero-discordant is a term used to describe a relationship in which one person is HIV-positive and the other is HIV-negative.

Daniel was still married to his husband, Mason, who was living back east and was moving ahead with divorce proceedings. Daniel professed to still be in love with Mason, but since he wanted to make Minnesota his permanent residence, divorce seemed to be inevitable. Despite his recent HIV diagnosis, Daniel was physically healthy. He was diagnosed as bipolar at age eighteen, however throughout his life, Daniel had resisted this diagnosis to the point of absolute denial. He would stop his medication, be seemingly fine for a while, and then would experience severe depression and/or mania. At age twenty, Daniel reported having his first sexual experience with a stranger in a motel. Daniel said no feelings were involved in this experience, but it "validated his gayness." In his mid-twenties, he was raped. He did not tell anyone, feeling too embarrassed to do so, and believing he "must have been asking for it." He began sexually acting out—and was drawn to the dominant/submissive subculture.

Daniel listed his stressors as: financial, being in a sober house, his impending divorce, being HIV-positive, and homesickness. This session began an "adventure" which continues to this day. I could never have anticipated the pain, sadness, worry, exhilaration, joy, and incredible learning experience that was to come. As I have told Daniel (to quote a line from the old song, "Thanks for the Memory,") "You may have been a headache, but you never were a bore." And, I would not have missed this therapist/client relationship for the world.

Kathy's Notes—July 8, 2008

Daniel went back to inpatient treatment in June 2008. When he was discharged, we begin therapy again. Daniel has moved in with a friend he made while in treatment who lives in Minneapolis. He states he has little will to live, which is very scary to hear. Daniel told Mason to proceed with divorce proceedings, and this was a very difficult decision. He has started attending a sexual health group in his outpatient group, and has made a commitment to remain celibate for at least ninety days, and afterwards, he will re-evaluate his decision at the group and in our therapy sessions. Daniel talks about feeling "like a chameleon," and hates the behavior associated with this. A recurring theme for Daniel is *trying to be what he perceives other people want him to be.*

July 22, 2008:

Daniel will move into his own apartment next Monday. While he was at his last sober house, something very significant happened. Daniel had about a month of experiencing flu-like illness during his sero-conversion process, and slept almost constantly. When the house manager confronted him about his being in bed so much, Daniel divulged his HIV-positive status. The manager insisted Daniel reveal this news to everyone in the house. The manager threatened that Daniel would be discharged from the house if he did not comply, so Daniel did.

I was appalled when he told me this. We shared this information with Daniel's case manager at Minnesota AIDS Project (MAP), whose reaction was the same. The attorney at MAP was consulted, and although Daniel opted not to look into legal proceedings against the sober house, he wanted the owner and staff to become educated about the rules of privacy when it comes to HIV status.

The documentation of this time truly points out how serious and important it is for people to have a right to privacy when it comes to their healthcare, and any related issues. Since the passing of HIPAA laws, every American is briefed about the act when seeing any new health care professional or service. HIPPA refers to the American Health Insurance Portability and Accountability Act of 1996, and it is a set of rules to be followed by doctors, hospitals, and other health care providers. HIPAA helps ensure that all medical records, medical billing, and patient accounts meet certain consistent standards with regard to documentation, processing, and handling of all health-care information. Significant numbers of laws, both federal and by the states, also protect people from the stigmas of having HIV or AIDS, as well as most other health concerns. The reason for these laws is to protect people from being unjustly discriminated against by others who find out about a given illness.

Up until the 1980s, we do not know how many people developed HIV or AIDS. HIV was unknown, and people didn't know the signs/symptoms of transmission. According to www.avert.org/professionals/history-hiv-aids/overview:

- While sporadic cases of AIDS were documented prior to 1970, available data suggests that the current epidemic started in the mid- to late 1970s.
- By 1980, HIV may have already spread to five continents (North America, South America, Europe, Africa, and Australia). In this period, between 100,000 and 300,000 people could have already been infected.
- In 1981, cases of a rare lung infection called Pneumocystis carinii pneumonia (PCP) were found in five young, previously healthy gay men in Los Angeles. At the same time, there were reports of a group of men in New York and California with an unusually aggressive cancer named Kaposi's Sarcoma.
- In December 1981, the first cases of PCP were reported in 386 people who inject drugs. By the end of the year, there were 270 reported cases of severe immune deficiency among gay men—121 of them had died.

When HIV was first discovered and researched in the 1970s and 1980s, it was nothing short of terrifying. People who tested positive lost their jobs, became outcasts in society, were dropped from insurance carriers, and often faced losing even their closest family and friends due to fear and stigma. The same thing continues to happen in today's society, with a HIV or mental health diagnosis, along with various other diseases.

People often act and react out of fear. The monetary and civil damage affecting these people is often insurmountable, but finally the laws are catching up with the needs of the society, and everyone in it. We have a long way to go yet. Vast numbers of people continue to be terrified of these illnesses in their lives, and too often their fear, fueled by the stigmas still very much alive, prohibit people who need care and assistance from seeking it. Some people who know they may have been exposed to HIV, or have mental health issues ranging from bipolar disorder to clinical depression, and everything in between, don't seek professional diagnosis or care because the cost of this information being public is simply to high. Truly this is one of the main reasons for our writing this book together—to give the two perspectives.

Daniel's Work with Kathy

By owning, sharing, and reflecting on our experience together, Kathy and I hope it might help people become more educated about what these illnesses are truly about. By deciding to openly and honestly share the journey we have taken to understand these illnesses, and how they affected my life as a person, and Kathy's life as a professional caregiver and advocate, it might show that as scary as the process can sometimes be, it is not insurmountable. Perhaps this will help others who have or might have these diagnoses in their own life to find the courage and hope to come forward and get help themselves, without quite so much of the terror about whether they can be happier and healthier than ever before in their lives. Living with bipolar disorder, HIV, or the many other co-occurring challenges can be surmounted, but everyone faced with these challenges has to find his or her own answers and coping skills.

Kathy's Notes—August 1, 2008:

Daniel was a "no show." I left a message; this makes me very worried. It is unlike Daniel not to call and either cancel or reschedule if he cannot make an appointment.

August 7, 2008:

Daniel called and said his medication, Seroquel, was "knocking him out." He says he has done nothing but sleep for the past week, and has not been checking his messages.
NOTE: Seroquel is a brand name of the medication *quetiapine fumerate*. It

is classified as an antipsychotic medication, which means that it is used to try and restore the natural balance of neurotransmitters in the brain. It is primarily prescribed to treat people who have schizophrenia and bipolar disorder. Often the same medications are used to treat various mental health conditions even though the conditions themselves may be completely different. This is important to know so that no assumptions are made that include all symptoms of one illness also exist with another. Example: bipolar disorder and schizophrenia may have similar medications used in their treatment, but not because the illnesses are related.

Seroquel is an antipsychotic medication. It works by changing the actins/proteins of chemicals in the brain. It is used to treat schizophrenia in patients who are at least 13 years old, and adults and children who are over 10 years old who are bipolar. It is also used together with antidepressant medications to treat major depressive disorder in adults. For Daniel, Seroquel has been helpful in managing his symptoms of mania, especially if he can recognize the early signs and intervene before it escalates to a dangerous level.

August 15, 2008:
Another missed appointment. This time I called Daniel's psychiatrist, Dr. Jon Grant. He said he would decrease the Seroquel, and increase Daniel's antidepressant, Effexor.

August 18, 2008:
Daniel made it to today's appointment, but admitted to isolating himself much of the past couple of weeks. He signed releases allowing me to contact two of his close friends here in Minneapolis, in case he "disappears," or I am concerned. Both friends have keys to Daniel's apartment as another safety measure. Daniel said he feels like a failure in all areas of his life, the only exception being in his sex life, an area where he says he feels he is competent. He also says he feels being a satisfying sexual partner validates him as a gay man.

I encouraged him to begin journaling again, but felt pretty ineffectual at helping him feel better about himself. He struggles so with his bipolar diagnosis, his shame, his HIV status—and life in general. Whew, a heavy session, but I am so glad he came. One of the most important things I had to learn in this profession was how to care deeply for my clients, but be able to leave as much of the therapy work as possible in the office. It is a delicate balance and something I will continue to work on as long as I am doing therapy.

Chapter 9

Depression, Mania, and Medication

Medication for bipolar disorder is often best described as a necessary evil—because this is how it so often feels. Someone who has never had to rely on psychiatric care or medication may not realize why it is often such a battle taking these medications, or why so many people who do need them find themselves in a struggle to do so. As I have said already, I have had times of medication adherence, and times when I completely went off of my medications. My brain chemistry does not regulate my moods in the same way as a person without the disorder. It is not clear to this day what causes bipolar disorder. It is thought that genetics plays a role, but episodes can be brought on by extreme stress or physical changes. Equal numbers of men and women struggle with the disease, which is marked by extreme changes in moods. *Mania and depression are the two ends, or poles, of the spectrum.* Mania can present in many different ways, and manifests differently in different people. For instance, I can see my mania forming when my behaviors become more risky. Things like driving at higher speeds than usual, or finding myself unable to sleep at night, are common early-warning symptoms. Not all symptoms occur during every manic episode, and I am usually able to navigate mania without causing myself harm, but that has been only after extensive experience and hard work.

These are the major symptoms of mania that I have experienced:
- Restlessness
- Racing thoughts
- Euphoric happiness and feelings of elation
- Utopic sense of hope
- Sudden and severe irritability
- Anger, rage, and extreme hostility
- Poor concentration and inability to maintain attention
- Rapid speech and inappropriate commentary
- Surges of energy
- Inability to sleep as well as lack of being tired
- Impulsive behavior
- Insatiable sex drive
- Feelings and behaviors rooted in self-grandiosity
- Poor sense of judgment
- Drug and alcohol abuse

Depression is the other end of the spectrum, and for me it can usually be expected after a manic episode. Depression is another hugely misunderstood ailment in our society. Depression is not just being sad or feeling blue. Rather, it is the inability to change one's own subdued mood, accompanied by extremes in sadness and desperation. A truly depressed person will not be cheered up simply by slapping a smile on his face, and often will just blend in. Many people are walking around struggling with clinical depression that they keep totally secret, or let only their closest confidantes know. Depression lurks there silently, quietly destroying everything you care about with its paralyzing effect.

Following is a list of common symptoms of clinical depression:
- Extreme and unrelenting sense of sadness and hopelessness
- Lack of energy
- Loss of self-worth
- Loss of interest in things usually enjoyed
- Inability to concentrate or complete tasks as usual

- Irritability
- Extreme shifts in appetite, one way or another
- Excessive sleep
- Suicidal ideation/thoughts (passively fantasizing about suicide, or actively attempting suicide)

The tricky thing with this type of bipolar disorder is *treating mania without causing depression—and treating depression without causing mania.* You cannot just treat for the active symptoms, but rather have to medicate to try and bring balance between the two extremes. Once I get these chemicals to a state of balance, and start feeling better overall, it is not long until they become imbalanced again, and then it is back to the drawing board. Sometimes I have gone months without an episode of mania or depression, and sometimes I have had mania, depression, or a cycling back and forth between the two occur for months on end. There is no way to predict it, and I have found the best way to navigate it has been building a strong support structure of family, friends, and professionals.

Finding the Right Psychiatrist

This is why it is so very important to work with a psychiatrist whom you genuinely trust and believe in. It is equally important to work with a psychiatrist who never gives up on a patient. Some doctors I have seen have been ready to throw their hands in the air when so many medications have been tried and did not work, or stopped working. All too frequently these doctors blame the suffering party for not really trying when he is in fact, giving it his all. This is a deadly error, and in my opinion, if you ever have a doctor express this type of attitude towards your care, or *your* medication regimen, stop seeing this doctor immediately, and find one who has another idea. It should be criminal for a doctor to tell a patient there is nothing more to try or can be done. Proactive doctors are always willing to be honest with their patients, but are also open to new ideas and methods of treatment. The cocktail of medications that worked at one time might not be the cocktail that will work now. Some people find one medication regimen that will work for them for years, and that is wonderful. Generally my doctor and I have had to tweak dosages and medications frequently as my brain seems to adapt to one regimen, and then falls out of balance again, or some outside stressor elicits a relapse of symptoms.

This makes it easy to see why illicit drug use is so common among people with mental health issues. If I use crack cocaine, methamphetamine, or even alcohol, I know what the general result will be. I have some control over the result, even if it makes my behavior so out of control while under the influence. I was fortunate to find a psychiatrist who is willing to never throw in the towel. At times I have been ready to give up, but this doctor has never given up on my health—or me. He has never judged me for turning to illicit substances out of frustration or desperation, yet has repeatedly worked to help me find good medically approved substances. He also listens to me when I tell him something is not working. He is open to a phone or email consultation with me between our regular appointments. He works with and for me, and the mutual respect that we have for one another helps in our medical relationship. Remember, your doctor deserves your respect, but if he is not giving you the respect of his time and effort in return, get a new one.

This doesn't mean your doctor is your puppet, set to do what you want when you want. Sometimes my psychiatrist has had to tell me that I needed to give a medication more time, or even saying "No" to a medication I have requested because he knew it was not appropriate for my overall health. Trust is the key here. Be open and honest, and demand the same in return. The vast majority of doctors and healthcare nurses want to help, so find those caregivers. When you do, you must be willing to be vulnerable, trusting, and honest with them. Otherwise, the only person who gets hurt is you.

Sometimes medications I have been on have made me feel like a zombie. Medications, especially psychiatric ones, often have challenging side effects. Weight gain, sweating, bloating, headaches, nausea, diarrhea, and tiredness are a few of the many side effects I have experienced over the years. My doctor and I decide together when they are too much, and move on to something else. Some of the side effects I have learned to live with over time, and others I simply could not accept. Some of my current health concerns have been caused by the use of certain medications in the past. For instance, my liver suffered damage as a result of using the drug Depakote as a mood stabilizer.

The bottom line is to have a working relationship. I never give up on new options, and my doctor has proven he will never give up on me. Unfortunately a vast number of people are not able to find this quality of help in the care of their mental health. When my doctor moved his practice from Minneapolis to Chicago, and because I believe in the work we do together so much, we set up a system to work with each other, which may not always be the most convenient, but it is worth it to maintain the relationship with this doctor who I wholeheartedly trust.

Also realize that many factors can change the effectiveness of medication—weight loss or gain, seasons, diet, etc. Meds work better or worse at times for many reasons, some are medical and others are environmental. Attitude, perspective, and your support structures change, and having a psychologist to keep up to date and explore these changes with is invaluable.

When I have great stress in my life, my symptoms are generally worse. I am wonderful in a crisis, but afterwards it takes me some time to get back a sense of balance. I notice major changes in my mood when the seasons change. The different amounts of UV light I am exposed to effects my moods. I always know when we have a full moon, which I find very humorous. I guess one might call me a "lunatic." Consider this: The moon controls the tides of the oceans, and as the human body is made up of almost entirely water, we should not be surprised that the lunar cycle affects our moods. Sometimes the answer is not changing the medication, but having a healthy support system in place to navigate those challenging times not within our own control. It is helpful to have a good sense of humor about the one thing we all have in common: our humanness.

Chapter 10

Religion and Spirituality

Kathy's Notes—August 2008:
Daniel went back to inpatient treatment for help with his chemical dependency. I saw him weekly while he was there. He continued to talk about the pain of his divorce, and how the marriage represented "success" to him. Daniel has also come to realize that in his mind, getting married was the "best chance of getting acceptance from his family."

Ironically, not everyone in Daniel's family was able to accept Daniel's marriage as legal, thus his dream of acceptance was not realized. Daniel was stuck in the "it's all my fault" mode during the duration of his stay at inpatient treatment. He stated that he felt like a failure as a gay man and a husband. No amount of reassurance on my part helped.

In hindsight, I should have known better. This was Daniel's reality, and only he could move past it. A recurring lesson professionally and personally is just being there, and being present to Daniel and all of my clients is often, or maybe always, *enough*. I cannot take the pain away as much as I might like to. Perhaps a better lesson is to help people endure pain without bringing more on themselves by making bad choices. A quote, usually attributed to Buddha, says, "pain is inevitable—suffering is optional."

The *meaning* of pain is a great discussion topic, for individuals and/or groups. If pain is something to be avoided, to what lengths will a person go in order to do this? If it is inevitable, is there value in it? *Growing pains* implies that with pain there is almost always growth, and that is valuable.

For me, the best example of this is childbirth. Anyone experiencing it will readily agree that it is painful, but this pain culminates in the creation of a new human being.

September 2, 2008:

Daniel is seeing Dr. Grant weekly because he feels down and depressed. What may be exacerbating this is the fact that Daniel is working on his fourth step in his 12-step recovery program where there seems to be a huge emphasis on his "defects of character." While the philosophy of the fourth, fifth, and sixth steps of the 12-step model is sound, to ask a depressed, shame-based person to dwell on his "defects" is counter-productive and potentially harmful.

Daniel identifies himself as the "black sheep" of his family. We are working very hard to help him shed this identity, not reinforce it. During this session, Daniel engaged in very degrading self-talk. He was not only self-critical, but resentful towards God (doubting God's existence and most certainly that God could be a "loving God"), toward authority figures, and Mason's mother. Daniel believes she was influential in encouraging Mason to divorce him, and she pressured Mason to make this decision, and not entirely of his own volition.

Daniel's attitude toward the existence of God was so conflicted. What if he did not believe in God's existence? Would it mean Daniel was certain to go to hell? I am always puzzled by a person who professes to be an atheist or agnostic—but at the same time, has such strong feelings about God. Not only allowing but also encouraging the client to express these feelings is a unique experience, because the usual response is to keep them secret—and then feel guilty about having such feelings.

As a strong Catholic, I keep my belief system private unless a client wants to engage in a discussion about religion and/or spirituality. I have found the best approach is to support the client's opinion about God, and let the client be free to change or alter this as he goes through the process of therapy. It was not Daniel's disbelief that was disturbing to me, but rather his idea that if he somehow *did not do "the right thing,"* he was sure to be punished for all of eternity.

Daniel's Insights

This is a very good place to comment on the spiritual part of my story. I was raised in a very devout Irish Catholic family. In my teenaged years, I thought I might become a Roman Catholic priest one day, or at the very least, hold some role within the Catholic Church. I am no longer a Catholic. I never thought I could find a spirituality I could believe in my heart and soul, and still be a member of a devout Catholic family. I appreciate with my entire self the gift of faith that was instilled in me by my parents. It was not always easy for us to reconcile my leaving the Catholic Church, and choosing instead to believe in a spirituality that sometimes conflicts with Catholic doctrine. I believe I was genetically born as a homosexual, and also that I was created spiritually as a homosexual. I do not accept that my sexuality was a mistake of nature or a disorder of some sort. I believe that we exist in human form to experience life, and to learn lessons of the soul.

> **I believe we are all a part of a greater whole, that the whole is one of goodness and love, and that pain and suffering help us to evolve into stronger, greater beings.**

I believe in evolution, and respect creationism as a theory of human existence, developed in a time when there was not the science we have today. I support spiritual texts as tools of perception, be it The Bible, The Quran, the Gnostic Gospels, etc. I am not a literalist and I do not think any text or any spiritual book is an absolute truth. I vehemently oppose using such texts as means of condemning other people. I sometimes attend liberal churches when I feel I need the support spiritually, but have not yet felt an obligation or desire to join a church. I believe hell is something that is experienced when our hearts, minds, and souls are disconnected from God and others. It is a space devoid of love and goodness. I do not believe in a fiery pit of punishment.

The only hell I have experienced happens enough here in this lifetime and in this human form. I believe that souls evolve, and that souls who persecute and harm others are severely disconnected. An eye for an eye seems to me to be a human tool of punishment, not a spiritual one. I struggle with this at times when I encounter true evil. I believe I am a work in progress on every plane of energy. I believe myself to be a soul maturing, rather than one sinning. I believe in metaphysics, and that we all are divine expressions of God: single parts of one great energy whole. I know one thing for certain: I will never in my human form have the ability to prove concretely or scientifically who or what God is. I believe in the golden rule of Jesus Christ: to do unto others, as I would have others do unto me, and I try imperfectly to follow this rule. I do not believe that it is a uniquely Christian idea but rather one that is expressed in most faiths, just in different ways. Although I think the story of Jesus is a wonderful expression of the power, strength, and love that is God, I do not believe that the mystical lessons therein are dependent on any historical accuracy of details.

I may or may not discover an absolute truth after I die. Whatever the case, I believe God, the Universe, Allah, Buddha, and all other gods from all other religions throughout history have value and deserve respect. Truly God can be seen and felt dwelling in any manifestation of life. My spirit *rejoices in not knowing*. The past is something to learn from. The future is something to be revealed in its own due time. The *now* is all I have any influence over through the choices, perceptions, attitudes, and level of mindfulness with which I approach it. My life is an opportunity to connect with the people, the world, and the life surrounding me, and I support life and experience with all the love of my heart and mind.

Today, my family and I respect one another's belief systems, as well as our right to have our own belief systems be paramount. We are all being mutually respectful of one another's beliefs and boundaries, so there is no tension when we are together. My mother is the most devoted person I have ever known. Her faith and the love of her children and grandchildren are traits of which I am constantly in awe. Because she has had the courage to stand by her convictions in life, even when it was not the easy thing to do, I have that same courage within me. I take responsibility for my actions and reactions, and I stand up for what I believe in, publicly and proudly. I may not agree with another person's beliefs or opinions, but I will never abandon the fact that he has a right to them as much as I have a right to mine. If being right is more important to anyone than being at peace with one another, we will always have holy and political wars. Nothing is worth that, nothing. This is my spirituality, and it effects every decision I make. Everything we do, say or express into the world has both a cyclical and rippling effect.

Chapter 11

Watching His Words

Kathy's Notes—September 9, 2008:

Daniel began the session by saying "Life is hard. My will to live is not there." I want my clients to tell me how they really feel, but sometimes hearing what they say can be *so hard*, and this is one of those times. A lot of discernment is necessary when working with fragile and seriously depressed clients. When Daniel said he didn't have the will to live, I did not immediately conclude that he was suicidal, but of course I needed more information. As the session continued, Daniel was clear in that he had no immediate plan for self-harm, but was in a very dark place as a result of some dreams and recent manic behavior. Daniel relates disturbing dreams, including one in which he is murdered. Daniel says he is afraid of hurting his friends and family because "that's what I always do." A very old friend called him, and he committed to return her call.

I am trying to keep him connected to people who have been his friends in the past. Daniel feels guilty about "not getting better." I encouraged him to explain this feeling to Dr. Grant. Knowing Dr. Grant professionally, I have faith that he will be able to offer Daniel some solace with these feelings, in addition to a possible medication change. Daniel talked about holding in anger to the point of being afraid of it. He feels his anger is too explosive and raging to express. Daniel is still saying, "I deserve to be HIV-positive, and to be bipolar." This statement came after he admitted he has been acting out sexually as a part of his manic phase. I continuously try to help Daniel change his word choices when it comes to his illnesses. It is important for him to accept that he has these illnesses, but it is equally important for him not to believe his entire identity is of being an addict, being bipolar or being HIV-positive.

> **Kathy: I remind Daniel that he is a person who has bipolar disorder, HIV, and chemical dependency issues—but this is his behavior—not his identity.**

Daniel's Response

One of the most effective tools I learned through the therapeutic process with Kathy is to be conscious of my word choices and have integrity to stand by what I say. Lying comes in many forms, and I have in the past been a very good liar. I lied to hide things, and I lied to avoid things and feelings. I have also lied to myself, creating a person out of those lies that was not an accurate portrayal of who I really am. Sometimes when we continually proclaim something to be true, we make it true. This works both ways. It can create wonderful things and help us achieve our dreams, and it can work in a negative way that holds us back from evolving to a new level. The more I said, *I am HIV-positive, I am bipolar or I am an addict*, the more disgusted I would become with myself. This constant practice of reminding myself, and the world around me, that I was all of these things challenged my ability to build any genuine self-esteem, and it precluded me from being able to see myself as anything but a damaged and incomplete person.

I've always had issue with one of the main tenets of the 12-step system of recovery. At the start of 12-step meeting, everyone introduces themselves with their name and the statement, "I am an addict," or "I am an alcoholic," or "I am a sex addict." I can understand the rationale behind making this statement is to remind oneself that addiction is one acting-out behavior away from being completely destructive again. However, it can also reinforce this idea that the person actively pursuing a life where he doesn't allow these behaviors to control him can never *actually* get away from these behaviors. This is my opinion and feeling on the matter.

For a long time, and through hundreds of meetings, I introduced myself this way: "Hi, my name is Daniel, and I am an addict." After a couple of years, I changed to, "Hi, my name is Daniel, and I am a grateful addict." Now I never refer to myself as an addict. I have been able to stop seeing myself as addicted; instead I see myself as being empowered by choices. I am not denying that I am very susceptible to addictive behavior and substances. I do not deny that addiction and its ensuing behaviors can seem impossible to overcome. I do however believe in the ability to recognize the difference that empowerment makes.

This minor change may not seem like much, but, for a person like me who is constantly in a state of vigilance over keeping my mental awareness in balance, *it makes a world of difference.* Sometimes people who were new to a meeting would come up to me at the end and ask me why I identified myself differently. After I explained, most often I was met with a sense of respect and awareness—and this works best for me, because it is more than acceptable to do what is best for me and my health.

Using Electroconvulsive Therapy (ECT)

As I explained earlier, sometimes the medication used to treat bipolar disorder doesn't work as well as is needed to maintain stability and functionality in my life. It is these times when it helps a lot to be open-minded to new ideas surrounding possible treatments. My psychiatrist brought to the table Electroconvulsive Therapy (ECT). ECT has been around for decades, but the first connotation that might come to mind is of being strapped to a chair, and zapped by some sort of torture device. This may have more closely resembled what it once was, but it is not the experience I had when using ECT as a form of treatment today. The treatment itself takes place on either an outpatient or inpatient basis. Patients who are checked into a psychiatric care ward at a hospital often find it helpful to be there, as it is more convenient, and they have constant supervision during the process. However, hospitalization is not necessary, which pleased me because I have gone out of my way not to be hospitalized unless absolutely necessary.

The procedure, including recovery time, commonly took the better part of a morning, four to five hours. A targeted electronic pulse is delivered to a specific area of the brain. This application jumpstarts the brain's chemistry in order to improve the release of mood chemicals. Afterwards I mostly remember being tired more than anything, and usually the remainder of the days when I had these treatments, I spent sleeping and resting.

I used ECT on an outpatient basis, having a friend come with me for every treatment. Treatment generally is given three times a week, with a day of rest in between each session, but some people are treated frequently, varying every five days, or once a month. A typical treatment looks something like this. After checking in, the patient is evaluated about what he experiences side-effect wise, and whether he has had any improvement of depression symptoms. Next, the patient is placed on a gurney where any needed medications and anesthesia is given so the patient is asleep during the procedure. It takes only a few minutes to receive the treatment, but I always woke up and was transferred to a wheelchair before I was consciously aware I was awake. Sometime while sipping juice at the nursing station, I would realize I was awake, and I never quite got used to my experience, so I just laughed at it.

I had some success with ECT. I tried it on three separate occasions, receiving about fourteen treatments in each set. I did experience memory loss, and to this day have some struggles with word recall during conversations. I also have trouble cementing some new memories. This is most noticeable when I watch movies or read books. I can remember all the movies I saw before my ECT, but when I watch a movie since having the treatments, within a few days I will forget what the movie was all about. Even this can be fun. I can watch great movies over and over, and it is like I am seeing them for the first time.

These experiences can sometimes be frightening and a little surreal. It is much more helpful to find humor in it than to dwell on the unknown rationality of it. The greatest mentors I ever had in life were a couple who lived across the street from me where I grew up. Bob and Claire were about fifty years old when I was born, and they had raised six children, some of whom babysat for my brother and me when we were little. Bob and Claire offered a safe port in the storm. I would go across the street every night while in high school. I would go the same time every night, before my homework and after dinner. It was a chance to get away from the turmoil of my mind before I had sought help for the bipolar disorder when I was eighteen. We would watch *Wheel of Fortune* and *Jeopardy* together, and I would often share glimpses of myself that I was not comfortable sharing with everyone else.

Claire taught me that life was a steady stream of change, and accepting and evolving with this change was going to be easier than dwelling on the way things used to be, or how I wanted things to be. Bob was the most optimistic person I have ever encountered. He had one response to what may be life's most common question. Whenever anyone asked Bob, "How are you?" Bob would reply in an enthusiastic voice, "Outstanding!" I can still hear his booming voice saying this, even though he died a few years ago. This sense of optimism, no matter how good or bad things may have been at the time, formed the cornerstone of the perspective I live life with today.

No matter what else is happening in life, each person has the ability to choose his or her own perspective. Sometimes I choose to be overwhelmed or negative, and as a result, I attract more negativity and chaos into my life. When I choose to be positive and careful about the thoughts and actions that I put into my brain and out into the world, I find the strength to take life as it comes with a faith that things will work out with time. I still don't have all the same emotions and challenges as I did before, but being conscious of the fact *I am not a bystander or a victim in my life, even when it feels like it,* I am empowered at every level of my being. In my heart this will always be a doctrine to live by, as best I can.

> **No matter what else is happening in life, each person has the ability to choose his or her own perspective.**

Kathy's Notes—September 30, 2008:

Daniel will have ECT on Friday because his current medication regimen doesn't seem to be effective. He also recently went to his infectious disease doctor, and his HIV blood work is as follows: T-Cells: 473, viral load: 71,000. His infectious disease doctor wants to wait six months before starting Daniel on any drug therapy in the hopes Daniel can first stabilize the bipolar disorder. Dr. Grant is suggesting long-term disability. Daniel is resistant, but has agreed to consider it. He states his biggest concern with this is the stigma surrounding being "disabled."

    Daniel says he has been a "shut in" for the past week, and he has been extremely depressed for the past three weeks. He also reports having even lost his interest in sex.

October 7, 2008:
Daniel has had two ECT sessions this week. He reports feeling "exposed," having a constant headache, extreme fatigue and short-term memory loss. He said he attended a 12-step meeting and feels he "doesn't fit in." Daniel said he is "dangling." I'm not sure what this means, but I am not interpreting this as *anything good*. So far, ECT doesn't seem to be helping, but Daniel will continue. Daniel will attend a new church. He is searching for spirituality in some church, group, etc. Daniel's brother, John, will be coming to visit in a few weeks. He will be here for only a day, but Daniel wants to be honest with him about being HIV-positive, and about his relapses. *This is a risk.*

October 14, 2008:
Daniel says ECT seems to be working better. He seems to have more energy, but is very angry—at God, himself, and the men who have degraded him sexually, especially during sex with drug use. Then Daniel said, "I don't have the right to be angry." This is a *big theme* throughout all of therapy with him. Anger has never been expressed in a healthy way as a model for him. I always try to reinforce the need to accept the anger, and express it in some way that's not destructive. If not, I am afraid Daniel will become more and more depressed.

    Once again, Daniel said, "I feel like a failure"—wonder if this is connected with his brother's upcoming visit? Daniel said, "My using makes me disconnected...I really need to be connected." There is so much self-deprecating talk, I sometimes wonder if Daniel can ever be aware of what *a wonderful person he is,* I know it's not enough to keep telling him this, so I don't, but I do feel helpless at times when he is in despair.

October 23, 2008:
Daniel's brother's visit was very "calming." Daniel said ECT "seems to be working," and his highs and lows (rapid cycling) are not as extreme. He is accepting that he is an "addict." I struggle with the concept that this is one's identity, but I know it is a tenet of 12-step philosophy. I much prefer looking at the chemical abuse as a behavior, but I don't feel this is the right time to discuss this with Daniel.

Daniel is accepting that his relationship with Mason is over. In fact, he sold his engagement ring and wedding band. Even so, we thought it would be wise to have a friend with him when he travels to Boston to sign the final divorce papers. Daniel said the last four days have been hard. He says he has been to and spoken at 12-step meetings each day, sometimes multiple times a day. Mood appears to be very good.

Daniel's Take on the Term "Chronic Relapser"
This is a term that is well known to everyone who has had some level of recovery from substance and other abuses in their lives. I hate this term. The connotation is always negative for someone labeled a "chronic relapser." It is not ever a productive label, and it is the perfect example of why we must, as a society, choose our words very carefully. I don't in any way claim to be perfect, and I certainly don't claim to practice this philosophy perfectly. I have stuck my foot in my mouth so many times I think sometimes I should stuff a sock into the gaping hole in the middle of my face. However, I try to be more conscious of what I say, and how I say it. Blanket judgments, and even classifications of things that for all intents and purposes are true, can still create a reality that can be devastating in the mind of a person who's in a state of progress.

My feelings of being a failure and a loser came back tenfold with every relapse I have ever experienced. Addictions are habits, which means they have a perfect memory. When I choose to pick up a mood-altering substance, I am immediately transported to the level of destructive behavior I had abandoned when I stopped using. However, there's great hope in this. When I stop using, or make a decision that the substance and behaviors associated with its use, although perhaps too powerful to overcome alone, is not too powerful to be overcome if I turn to a source of greater power than me alone—I am empowered. This empowerment picks up right where it was dropped when I decided to turn back to the old behavior. It is a basic law of physics; every action has an equal and opposite reaction. If I survive the weakness, no matter how weak it may be, I will be much stronger after I live through it. What matters most is that I never stop striving to know better and to do better. It is equally important to recognize I must own my behaviors, mistakes, and successes—and not to give them more value than as a part of this one life.

Chapter 12

Let's Talk About Sex, Shall We?

Kathy's Notes—October 2008:
Daniel has had a damaging relapse on meth, and has returned to inpatient treatment. When I look back at the last entry in my case notes, now knowing that Daniel had such a bad relapse soon after our last session, it becomes clear to me: Daniel's most vulnerable times for relapse are *when he is feeling good*. This is very important to remember moving forward when we meet again after he is discharged.

November 13, 2008:
Daniel has been discharged from inpatient treatment. He is returning to his Minneapolis apartment, but he plans to move back into sober housing, and give up his apartment by December 1. This is positive, as living alone doesn't seem to be the healthiest situation for Daniel. He has completed his latest course of ECT treatments, and will be attending outpatient treatment three times a week. He is also attending a sexual health group one night a week, along with daily 12-step meetings. Daniel's family has agreed to continue helping him financially, with the stipulation he must continue to make his health and the care he needs his number one priority.

Daniel has begun to express vague dissatisfaction with parts of the 12-step programs he is involved in, as well as his work with his current sponsor. It is not clear to him at this time why this is happening, as he likes his sponsor and the support he receives from the recovery community.

November 20, 2008:

Daniel is back in the sober living house where he lived when he first left inpatient treatment back in February of this year. His sexual health group is bringing up some huge issues for him. He said he "got angry and defensive" when the facilitator of this group called him a "sex addict." Daniel takes responsibility for his unhealthy sexual practices, but insists his core issue is his self-esteem. *I soundly agree.*

Once again, the labeling turns up: "sex addict" implies an identity, not a behavior, and cannot be construed as anything but negative and shaming. For Daniel, as for many meth users, their sexual activity/acting out is closely, sometimes totally, connected with their drug use. When not actively using meth, their sexual activity is not an issue. Daniel is receiving mixed messages regarding his sexual activity. A "rule" at his sober house is that a resident is not to have any sexual contact with another resident. The word rule is in quotes because Daniel said this was enforced erratically, and on a case-by-case basis.

Daniel has not had any sexual contact with anyone he lives with, or with anyone he has lived with in his history with sober housing. The mixed message is happening because his sexual health group approves of casual sex, and says this is a good practice in rebuilding one's values regarding sexual activities. Using the term casual sex means "hook ups," and having sex outside of a committed relationship. In my experience working with gay men, they are *quite adept* at having casual sex, and what they really need to learn is to develop *friendships* with men and women.

On his own, Daniel shared beginning his "plan" to start separating sexual activity from drug use. Daniel has decided to address his sexual needs through masturbation only. If he does decide to have any sexual partners, he insists that they be only mutually consenting in regards to what sexual activities are comfortable for both parties. I told Daniel his coming up with this new way of establishing his own sexual values is very positive and healthy behavior on his part. Daniel is committed to adhering to his plan, and re-evaluating it after a period of ninety days, as well as talking about it openly in therapy.

December 1, 2008:
Daniel has decided to work with a new sponsor, and this seems to be working out well as Frank is close to Daniel's age, and has a similar background when it comes to sex and drugs. Daniel has five months of continuous sobriety, which is his longest period to date.

Daniel Gives His Point of View About His Sexual Value System

Sex and sexual values play a very large role in most people's lives. Sex as a topic is often very uncomfortable for many people to talk, hear, or in this case, read about. This is understandable as there are many different viewpoints of sex and its appropriateness as a public topic. Anyone who knows me knows I don't have too much of an edit button, so to speak. I tend to speak my mind and my truth, and sometimes it can make people uncomfortable—and sometimes this can be a problem when connecting with people.

However, equally problematic can be *not* discussing something that's so much a part of every human experience. I am a man who is now very in touch with who I am as a sexual being. I own who I am, and I love that sex is a beautiful, enjoyable, and spiritual part of my life. I have had all kinds of sex—gay sex, straight sex, sex with multiple partners—you name it. Some of these sexual experiences were positive, and some were negative. However, because I was willing to openly and honestly talk about sex throughout the course of therapy, I was finally able to let go of any shame I had associated with my sexuality, or with sex itself. Now in my mid-thirties and married to an amazing man, I am able to have the most fulfilling and connected sex of my entire life. It took many mistakes and varying experiences to develop a sexual value system true to who I am.

My parents taught me the Catholic interpretation of sexual values—that only a man and woman who were married could have sexual relations as something that united the couple, and allowed for reproduction. I accepted this as my value system until I realized that it could not possibly fit for me. I was a man interested in having sex with other men. I also did not think that sex was a sin outside of the marital bed. I abandoned this philosophy and started my own explorations into sex and its meanings.

Intimacy and sex are very different things, but being able to unite the two, in whatever sexual relationship you may have in your life, is the most beautiful expression of passion and vulnerability I have ever experienced. Maybe you think you cannot relate to a gay man's sex life, especially mine, which includes these graphically honest details of a sexual history full of extremes. I suggest you can, and no matter who you are, this is another core similarity of the entire human experience. Sexual values are different for every person, and are also ever changing. Being honest about that when and where you feel it is appropriate, and in the fashion that feels right, you will help change sex from an activity that can trigger shame—to one of only love and human connection. If you are a heterosexual woman in your fifties, your sex life is going to look vastly different from mine. You might be thirty years into a marriage, or you might be divorced. You might be a man who is attracted to both men and women. Or, perhaps you find that the sexual fantasies you have, make you feel embarrassed when you even consider the idea of discussing them with someone else.

Whatever the case may be, I think we can all agree that sex should be all it can be. It is a wonderful part of being human, and nobody can write one rulebook on what is or is not appropriate in this area. I am constantly baffled by the extent to which religious and political affiliations impose "rules" about sex and sexual expression as if there is some black-and-white guideline to right and wrong.

In the past, I used sex as a means of self-degradation. That was harmful and disrespectful. When I have had sex with multiple partners at different times, and when I had sex with multiple partners at the same time, it was not unhealthy unless this degradation was present. I have had threesomes where all three of us were connected, and had a deeply moving and greatly enjoyable experience. Just because something may be different from what you know does not make it bad, it just makes it different. *Placing shame on sex is always harmful.* At the same time, knowing that your sexuality is a precious gift to be cherished and shared only with others whom mutually respect it is a huge part of having a truly fulfilling sex life.

Now that I am married to Brian, we have a shared sex life and sexual value system. It's not that we have all of the same desires or exactly the same views on sex, but we are united in this area of our lives, and we explore and respect each other's thoughts, feelings and actions regarding sex as two parts of one whole. He and I seem to have a deeper and deeper experience sexually all the time. What was great sex when we first started has become better than great in the years we have been together. We explore and enjoy each other, and our sex life is something we truly celebrate together. In no way do I think anyone has to have our sex life, just as we do not need to live by the rules of someone else's sexual value system. I can say one thing for sure: whoever declared that sex gets boring after marriage is not doing it right! My suggestion, for what it is worth, is this: Find someone you can truly trust to keep your confidence and be impartial, and for me, it was my therapist. Talk about who you really are, and I am sure sex will enter the conversation. Doing so will help you unlock your core sexual values and needs.

Having a healthy and happy sex life for anyone at any age is a positive and healthy part of life.

Chapter 13

The Letting-Go Process

One of the greatest lessons I learned through the therapeutic process was: *we let go of things when we are ready.* If I am holding onto a behavior or resentment, I am doing so because it brings me something valuable and necessary for my continued security, safety, or validation. When these old standbys in our lives start to cause us problems, it is usually time to assess whether or not they are perhaps outstaying their welcome, and thus time to let go of them with the respect they deserve, and move on to what works for us. Like my mentor/neighbor Claire told me, change is the only constant in life. My work with Kathy taught me how to effectively navigate change in my life, and to gracefully, and sometimes not so gracefully, let go of what no longer works, and try something new. This is true with all of the illnesses I face in my life. I am overall grateful for the lessons and experiences that being a man who is gay, HIV-positive, formerly addicted to drugs, with bipolar 1 disorder. Just looking at this sentence makes me chuckle, because I never expected to have any of those things in my life. Nonetheless, there they are and have been, and without them, I would not be the man I am today. What's more, they also help me to continually improve on myself.

I love myself, and I choose to take what I am given in life, and make it something great. Everyone has the same choice, every single day.

Owning one's *self* is in my opinion the most courageous and effective way to make life great, and to make the world a better place. However, it takes a lot of work, and as the case notes of my journey through therapy clearly show, I am not always very open to being accepted. What we hold onto is in essence a security blanket. To let go means we have something else to grab hold of. My friend Kate is a wonderful nurse who has had a great career. Recently she decided it was time to do something else, and went back to school to become a nurse practitioner. She decided she wanted something different, something more. It was hard for her to let go of the stability of her job, and grab onto the unknown of working and going to school for her advanced degree, but she did it anyway because she knew it was time. We all do this in different areas of life. Trying to make people be where we want them ignores and disrespects their comfort levels, and nobody ever changes unless they are in a place where they feel ready to do so.

> **I know if I meet someone where he is at,
> he is more likely to meet me where I am.**

Kathy's Notes—December 12, 2008:

Daniel's mood today is "okay." He is still experiencing major issues with fear, trust, and sadness. He is feeling emotionally supported by the other members of his sober house. The sexual health group is bringing up lots of heavy emotions. Daniel relates how at the time he would invite people to sexually assault him out of a strong need for punishment of some sort. At one time, he had been raped in a bathhouse by a male who had piercings. While telling me this story, Daniel said he could feel his mania increasing. I encouraged him to call his psychiatrist. Daniel complied, and Dr. G responded by increasing Daniel's Seroquel.

NOTE: Seroquel is an antipsychotic medication that works by changing the actins/proteins of chemicals in the brain.

Therapeutically, most times it is a judgment call how much a person should disclose during a session. While it is cathartic to deal with these significant memories in a safe setting, I could clearly see in Daniel's case, there was a risk of triggering either mania or depression if the memories became too painful. As much as therapy is a process that can be affected by outside or inside stimuli, so is bipolar disorder.

Lying and Other Behaviors
February 3, 2009:
Daniel still struggling with religious/spiritual questions, whether he is an atheist…or an agnostic. Seems to find comfort in his new church. Abilify® medication was added, but it didn't help for very long, so it was discontinued. The medication regime continues to be challenging, and changes frequently. Dr. Grant doesn't give up—and this gives Daniel hope.

NOTE: Abilify is a brand name for the medication aripiprazole, which is used in conjunction with other antidepressants to help balance and improve mood. It is in a class of medications called atypical antipsychotics. It works by changing the activity of certain natural substances in the brain. Abilify is indicated for the acute and maintenance treatment of mixed and manic episodes associated with bipolar 1 disorder. It is usually prescribed in conjunction with other anti-depressants and medications commonly used to treat bipolar 1 disorder. www.drugs.com.

We looked through the wedding album from Daniel's wedding to Mason. What a grand, over-the-top affair. Good to see Mason's mother and Daniel's father at last. It was bittersweet, knowing how quickly the "honeymoon" was over. Daniel has a bout of pneumonia, his first major illness since his HIV diagnosis. Physical illness often results in depression for HIV-positive people, and Daniel is no exception. Says he is down from eight to ten meetings a week to five.

February 9, 2009:
During the time when Daniel is attending Crystal Meth Anonymous (CMA), he realizes his sexual compulsivity *preceded his drug use*. And, the most significant new idea is that Daniel's mania manifests itself in self-destructive drug use, paired with unhealthy sex. It is fascinating to me how each client's bipolar mania manifests itself. I have one client who shoplifts "seriously" when manic, another woman who is delusional about relationships, believing casual acquaintances are in love with her. And, paradoxically, some people who are manic become totally convinced the bipolar diagnosis no longer fits.

More About My Experience With Clients Who Are Bipolar:

My very first experience with bipolar clients was in a juvenile sex offender program when I was doing my practicum. These adolescents—ages 13 to 18—had admitted to felony-level sex offenses such as sexual assault, rape, and incest. The majority of these boys had been diagnosed with Conduct Disorder or Anti-social Behavior. A child psychiatrist who I'll call Dr. D was convinced that these diagnoses were largely incorrect, and in fact, these boys had bipolar type 1 disorder. All staff who worked in the sex offender program had to keep detailed notes about the boys' behavior, mood swings, etc., and these results were discussed with Dr. D to determine if a bipolar diagnosis was accurate, and in the majority of cases, Dr. D's assumption was correct.

The second person who taught me about bipolar disorder was a client I met while a probation officer. David (not his real name) had come to court for several DWIs, had been to treatment, and was active in AA. That being the case, the judge ordered him to keep attending AA weekly and provide proof to me, the supervising probation officer. David was a middle-aged man, appeared very professional in demeanor and attire, and very willingly gave me the details of his story. He had been a successful insurance salesman, but was drinking very heavily. On several occasions, he would actually work non-stop for three or four days, and ended up selling more insurance in that time than anyone in the company's history. After this, he would literally collapse and be unable to get out of bed or function for several days. He would then start drinking to "come up," and the cycle would begin again.

> **Kathy: It is not at all unusual for undiagnosed bipolar people to try and regulate their mood swings by self-medicating.**

In treatment and at AA, he was told that this would all stop if he would just quit drinking. However, he did stop drinking, but continued to have these mood extremes. In his last treatment center, David started doing research on his own, and when he found a description of bipolar disorder, he knew this fit. He found a doctor who prescribed lithium, and that medication, combined with his sobriety, resulted in a new and very successful career in real estate.

One of my current clients, Helen (not real name), began seeing me after she had appeared in court for shoplifting for the third time. Her probation officer realized that Helen was not stealing out of need, but because of some emotional issue. Helen was forty-five at the time, single, lived with her mother on a large farm on the outskirts of Minneapolis, and was working as a medical technician. Helen was bright, educated, interested in horses, crafts, and travel, as well as her mother, aunts, cousins, nieces, and nephews. At one time, she had actually spent time in a women's prison as a result of numerous and serious shoplifting episodes. Helen would go for months without stealing, but then she would take something large or small—and always something she could easily afford.

After several years of this behavior, accompanied by periods of severe depression and anxiety, I suggested she see Dr. Grant, Daniel's psychiatrist. Dr. Grant ultimately diagnosed Helen with bipolar 1 disorder, and concluded that her periods of mania manifested itself by shoplifting. By prescribing the appropriate bipolar medication, Helen's moods became stabilized. I wish I could say that Helen never shoplifted again, but, just as in Daniel's case, her episodes were farther and farther apart (longest period of no shoplifting was three years), and the consequences were minimal. Again, like Daniel, these slips required medication adjustments, and of course therapy to look for any life events, thoughts or feelings that may have triggered the shoplifting. Whether it is with Helen or with Daniel—or any other bipolar client I work with—the client and I *always* learn something in the session following the incident.

Daniel's Thoughts On Impulsive and Compulsive

Imagine a word that defined something in between these two words—*impulsive* (noun, a sudden strong and unreflective urge or desire to act)—and *compulsive* (an irresistible urge to behave in a certain way, especially against one's conscious wishes). This is often exactly how my brain works. My natural action and reaction in life is to act from a place of emotion, or act on my feelings.

This doesn't mean I don't have any control over my actions or reactions, but it took a lifetime of mistakes in this area—followed by extensive therapy—to begin learning how to assess situations from a place that is logical as well as emotional.

Some might argue this book itself is an emotional purge of sorts, but it's not that at all. I say this because I have already written that book. At the age of nineteen, and while living in California, I decided to write an autobiography. At the time it was a wonderful achievement. I had put countless hours of work into it, and valued it because it was longer than two hundred pages. I finished the manuscript days before I moved back to my parents' home, and I printed out several copies, bound them by hand, and distributed them to family and friends upon my return. Then it was a way of proving to myself I could find some purpose in my decision to drop out of college and go "off script" on my life's journey.

I had so much to learn about myself, but I could not see it at the time. I just went full-steam ahead writing as if everything I was saying was true. In fact what I wrote back then was *more of what I wanted to be true.* I was still in tremendous pain, tortured by my emotional responses to everything in life. I was willing to do anything to have my pain validated, and although I had positive responses to the book, it was actually just written as another attempt to fit in, at least in my own mind. I wrote the book from the viewpoint of a chameleon, ever mindful of what were the areas where I thought others would find redemption.

Ultimately, if I could shock others, I thought impulsively that I would have a chance to be accepted, if only through means of some sort of pity. It was more important at the time to be accepted than to be honest. My only objective was to get a second chance at being "normal." This is a deadly road to travel. It did not take very long for this thought process to throw my newly establishing life into turmoil. My compulsions were in control. What I most wanted was to be *accepted by me*—and to own the person I was. Lying about that truth only brought more damage, because the truth always finds its way to the surface, and the story I had written about whom I was, was quickly tarnished for anyone who had their eyes open. When I revealed the actual truths about who I was, these truths were faced with confusion related to the others I had bared my soul in my writing, realizing my writing was not in fact true.

So what then is the point? There's one unifying force in all the different therapies I have tried: honesty. When I was nine years old, I began pathologically lying. I would lie about everything. I lied about whether or not I did my homework, to how I felt, and everything in between. The lies became so frequent I began to live in a world where truth was based on how well I could remember my lies. It did not make sense to me or anyone else at the time. I would lie bold-faced about things without any reason to lie. My mother could ask me if I remembered to brush my teeth, and I would say yes, even though I had not. This lie had no consequence, but I would tell it anyway.

My father asked me at the age of twelve if I had any desire to join a local football league, and learn how to play. I told him yes, even though I had no interest in football, and in fact playing a rough sport made me miserable. When tryouts started, and after pulling a lot of strings to get me into the league, I was so crippled by fear I had to quit. My father was livid. Had I said I did not want to play from the start, it would have been fine. The problem: I made a commitment to enroll, and it was not easy to get in the program. Suddenly I was breaking the commitment, allowing my fear and anxiety to prevail.

My father is a man of incredible integrity. It is actually one of the most admirable traits both my parents have. That being said, they really struggled with my frequent inability to follow through with my commitments. My parents taught me that my word was my bond, and it was invaluable for me to stand by it. It took me a long time to learn this particular lesson in life, but since I have, I understand.

These examples are two of the scores of lies I began telling at that early age. A pattern began to form, and lasted throughout my teens, and even into a long stretch of my twenties. So why the lying? Today it makes sense.

When the lying started, something else started. My sexual being encountered adolescence. I was sexually attracted to males, not females, which was not acceptable then, and in my mind it made me *abnormal and unacceptable*. Thus, the lies confused everyone so much my sexuality issue was never even addressed, and it became easier to hide. The lying was compounded as my brain became bipolar, and never was any worse than when I was using illegal drugs to self-medicate the pain.

Now in my thirties, I am blessed to be in a place of acceptance of myself just as I am. Life still presents similar challenges, but I take life on its own terms, and I work out solutions for my life based on a solid, honest integrity. This took a lot of courage, hard work, and practice. At times I still face hatred of who I am based on ignorance. I encounter people frequently who have prejudice against homosexuals. These people are often genuinely kind to my face, perhaps not realizing I know about their hateful talk about homosexuals, and me in particular.

When it became public knowledge that I am HIV-positive, this intensified. One woman I know, after she found out, actually pushed me back when I tried to hug her. This was incredibly hurtful. Over time that feeling has evolved to me no longer being invested in having a relationship with her. I even feel sorry for her ignorance, and it is a loss to both her and me that we cannot have a real relationship. People talk…and when I hear someone say something negative about me, it hurts. Then I let the pain go, reinforce that I am being true and honest to myself—and others, and move on. The only person who gains anything from the hate is the hater, and what he or she gains, I don't want.

Being in touch honestly with our own human condition is the strongest building bone of a person's integrity. When I own myself, the people who don't like who or what I am, distance themselves, and others are shown how powerful it is to be honest, open, and loving to themselves, thus changing the world around them for the better. Getting to this place, which is truly a happy and peaceful place to be, takes time and effort. You have to face the fears in order to overcome them. Sometimes the same fears come time and time again. The trick is to never be content in one's own evolution.

I can grow and learn as long as I am willing to keep working at knowing better…and doing better.

Lying can be both impulsive and compulsive. So can any other behavior. Behaviors are not out of our control, and we can always change a behavior if we choose.

Chapter 14

Shame-Based Feelings

Kathy's Notes—February 9, 2009:
More turmoil. Patrick, a sober-house resident, relapses, as does Daniel's sponsor, Frank. John, another resident is bingeing and purging, and another friend calls Daniel "aggressive," and stops speaking to him. Good news. Daniel's sex drive is coming back, but the *bad news* is he decides to "test himself" by going to a cruising park late at night to see if he can be strong if sexual advances are made. When he told me this, it resulted in a heavy conversation about how risky this was. I tried to convince Daniel that the world will offer many chances to be tested—and he doesn't have to *seek out* these opportunities. The great thing about Daniel is that when I come on pretty strong, he gets the point. This also validates my belief that we can use a form of confrontation with the client only if a strong therapeutic alliance has been established. Whew! Crisis averted, for the moment, anyway. We now laugh about Daniel's occasional urges to "test himself," and simply refer to the earlier "Loring Park incident."

February 17, 2009:
Daniel said he acted out on a phone line, and did sex, but no drugs, which is another risky situation. He "beat himself up" over this, and stayed in bed all day except to attend a Sex Addicts Anonymous meeting. Although Daniel felt awful about this, in my opinion, this was a positive experience, because it broke the bond between sex and drugs. A very wise psychol-

ogist consultant told me "What is wired together is fired together," and truer words were never spoken, especially in regard to sex and meth.

Daniel coming down *so hard* on himself when he hits a rough spot is an ongoing issue we discuss. As our therapy progresses through the years, it is gratifying to see how the harm-reduction philosophy about not catastrophizing events will ultimately help Daniel take responsibility for his actions, without demoralizing him. A recent increase in antidepressants pushed Daniel into mania, so this was decreased, but he stayed on Seroquel.

This is another example of the delicate balance of medications that must be constantly monitored. Daniel's mania often begins with self-destructive thoughts, along with very little sleep, high energy and extreme restlessness/anxiety. Daniel is stressing out about telling Patrick, whom he is dating, that he is both HIV-positive *and* bipolar. No matter how long a person has been diagnosed with HIV, one of *the* biggest concerns is, "When do I tell?" Some people prefer to tell on the first date, others wait until things start getting serious, and others will only date other HIV-positive people. It is a totally individual choice, and even one person's choice may change from time to time. A local organization, Minnesota Aids Project, has a "Disclosure Group" which helps men discern how and when to tell others their HIV-positive status.

In this session Daniel said in his dreams, he is "letting go of rage." Once again Daniel's struggle with accepting his feelings emerges. While he feels he is in control of his thinking, Daniel's feelings continue to plague him. As mentioned previously, anger was rarely expressed in a healthy way in his life, so it is no wonder this emotion causes such conflict, and even shame.

February 26, 2009:
Daniel was asked to be "trusted servant" at his AA meeting. Even so, Daniel feels "less than," and, "I can't give myself a break," and continues to set unrealistic expectations for himself.

March 5, 2009:
Oddly, Daniel started smoking cigarettes while in treatment, a common occurrence as so many people in early recovery seek alternatives to their old

chemicals of choice. His weight is up to 226 pounds, much of this as a result of his medications. Daniel is unhappy about his appearance—not a surprise, since I have often said 90 percent of all gay men think they are overweight. The serious part of this is that meth is one "quick-and-dirty" way to lose weight, and I have seen many men relapse to use meth again for just that reason. His HIV numbers are very good, which is encouraging. No meds prescribed for HIV yet, but maybe in a month. Daniel tried to open a checking account, but was told he couldn't until his divorce was final.

March 12, 2009:
Cancelled at the last minute. Daniel rarely does this, but I know when he does he is seriously depressed, and literally can't leave the house.

Daniel's Thoughts on Guilt, Shame-based Feelings—and Rage

The most destructive "feeling" to my self-esteem is now and has always been *shame*. My shame started early on in my life, from the time I knew I was sexually attracted to males, and I suppressed it because I was aware something seemed wrong about it. My shame started as most shame does, from guilt. As the guilt continues on unabated, and digs into a place of secrecy more and more deeply, it becomes shame. There, in the very pit of my subconscious, it meets another deadly emotion: rage. My rage was the result of unexpressed anger. Being angry about something is normal and healthy, while not expressing anger will cause it to fester beneath the surface, and turn into rage. For some reason, I did not know how to express anger, nor did I have a healthy example to model. Rage is also a common symptom for people with bipolar illness, causing serious overreactions. Add in the element of fear, and you have a perfect storm.

The shame and rage that continued to build incrementally in my psyche was driven by fear. Fear of being honest about who I was, and what I felt. I feared my secrets would be revealed, and at the same time, fearful they *would not be*. All of this fear-based shame and rage reached a point of no return with my array of health concerns. I was now HIV-positive, bipolar, addicted to drugs, and seeking Social Security disability.

All of these challenges in life come with a huge amount of stigma and a bigger concern than ever was that of self-worth. I had always been trying to fit in, and I was a person who did anything but fit in, more and more so with the mounting challenges that became a part of my life. My feelings are very strong about my inadequacy as a person, and the lack of acceptance in our culture about these issues. Many people are not well educated about these issues, and as a result, stereotypes become the default mode of thinking related to others struggling with these issues. Because these feelings of shame and rage were in this constant cycle, for a long time I attributed them solely to the bipolar disorder.

The brain of someone with bipolar disorder is often plagued by what is called *rapid cycling*. This refers to the often quick and unpredictable mood swings. I can wake up feeling happy and lighthearted some days, and any simple inconvenience will cause an over-exaggerated reaction in my brain chemistry. Any feeling of contentment can quickly be replaced by an overall sense of total doom and failure. The event doesn't have to be something big. Often it can be as simple as forgetting to do something, or getting a bill I was not expecting.

When I am in a place of good balance, I can handle life on its own terms and keep things in perspective. However, if my brain has an imbalance of mood chemicals, my reactions are often impulsive, and not appropriate to the situation itself. I have greatly benefited from learning how to recognize feelings but not react to them. If I give myself a little time with any given situation, I tend to make better decisions as to how to react to it. I try to be very mindful, and think before I speak. It is often less important to be heard than it is to understand what is actually being said, and why.

With HIV, it is a feeling that somehow you deserved the infection and the illnesses it causes because you are some sort of deviant. Thoughts like, "if only I hadn't slept around or been so stupid to use drugs" made me feel like I was asking for it, or that I was suffering the wrath of a vengeful god. Some people are still afraid to touch or even know someone with HIV or AIDS, and because it is scary, they seem to benefit from showing compassion to the infected person.

The stigma of drug addiction involves the idea that willpower is the only thing needed to overcome chemical dependence. While I agree that every use is a choice, it does not mean that people have the tools necessary to be able to choose not to use. The answer we turn to far too frequently is either a rehab center or prison, and neither option has a very good success rate. Most addicts and alcoholics don't want to put themselves or their families and friends through the horrors caused by their addiction.

In 1971, President Richard Nixon decided it would be a good idea to declare a "war on drugs" in this country. Today, substance abuse is seen as a choice by the lawfully disobedient. The war of drugs has made drug addiction more difficult to overcome as it casts all who find themselves addicted placed in the category of being a felon. Look at how poorly prohibition worked in the 1920s. Many times people do commit crimes while under the influence of substances, and this is inexcusable.

Treating the addiction itself as criminal is just putting a bandage on the problem. Many people are serving harsh mandatory sentences for drug use and abuse, and the punishment of prison is doing nothing to address the actual behavior that preceded the crime. Ignoring the core problem of the active addict—and ultimately exacerbating the addictive behavior to a place of deeper secrecy and shame—just breeds more of the same behavior. If these are the casualties of the war on drugs, then how will we ever win it? Issues like poverty, racism, sexism, lack of access to good medical care, and many others, go unaddressed, and we just end up with a bunch of pissed-off addicts being ushered back into society without proper coping skills or any incentive to do any better.

We treat marijuana differently from oxycodone because we have been brainwashed into thinking one is a prescription medication, which makes it okay, while the other is an illicit drug. Even though oxycodone is far more abused than marijuana—and its devastating effects reach further into the fabric of our society—it was not on the condemned list because it was prescribed. Every day I take a fistful of medications for my ailments. If I don't take them, people would say I am being irresponsible, but if I told those same people I smoke marijuana to treat my bipolar episodes and anxiety attacks, I would likely be condemned for that. Well, so be it. We are not making sensible choices or finding sensible solutions in the area of chemical health in this country…and we have to do better, and fast.

Kathy's Comments—March 17, 2009

Daniel just told his mom he has been smoking. He is trying to cut down, rather than quit completely. We talked about his pattern of lying, which he thinks began at age nine. He would lie to his mother and the teacher about doing his homework. He knew he was gay even then, and *wanted people to ask him* what was wrong. He has had five months of sobriety, and says he has been completely honest. His image is, "I'm a nice guy," which may be okay, but what happens when he isn't a nice guy?

People are so multi-faceted. How they see themselves, and how others see them, can sometimes be radically different. What is true for many gay people is that they are shame-based due to feeling "less than" from an early age. To counteract this, gay men may try to be "better than"—by being nicer, smarter, funnier.

To further compound this, Daniel has been afraid of his anger. He is aware that anger was expressed inappropriately in his family as both a cultural and generational pattern, and rather than show his anger, Daniel denies it and instead reverts to the "nice guy" image. When Daniel has talked about being treated disrespectfully by friends or family, I have learned to say something like, "Wow, that would really make me angry." The goal is to give Daniel permission to express his real feelings, and then decide if any action needs to be taken.

It is often difficult for clients to speak honestly about their parents because they feel this is a betrayal. As a therapist, I have to then explain that this is not about blame, but making sense of the client's feelings and behaviors. People want to know they're not "crazy," and when you can point out that, "Of course you feel that way, it's how you've been programmed," it will make sense. Daniel said he felt betrayed by his marriage vows, and understands Mason's love was conditional. Because Daniel wasn't getting his needs met by Mason, it's one reason he turned to drugs. Obviously, this is much more complicated, but that's what Daniel is saying today.

Daniel begins dating Brian, who is in another sober house. He and

Brian start out slowly, first having coffee; then spending part of the day together. I asked him to talk about what each of them wants in a relationship. Both Brian and Daniel are from the East Coast, and had come to Minnesota for treatment: Daniel for chemical dependency to crack and meth, and Brian, for alcohol.

Clinical Comments:

It amazes me that so many couples never discuss relationship expectations. Because I practice from a Humanistic-Existential base, I think it is important to discuss the meaning of things—especially issues like sex, commitment, family, and relationships. As an example, often after a couple has been together many years, they will realize sex means entirely two different things. For one person, it is sacred, and only to be done in the context of a committed relationship, and for the other person, it may only mean a physical release and need, with no emotional attachment.

Daniel's Thoughts:

Every event in our lives has one constant: perspective. Throughout most of my life, up until I entered therapy with Kathy, I generally held on tight to the past, and resisted change. My dear friend, Claire, saw this in me, which is probably why she so often talked to me about being able to accept change, and go with life's flow. I caused myself so much pain throughout the years by struggling to hold onto the way things once were, instead of trying to find the blessings and opportunities in the way things were yet to be.

> **I lived most of my life in the past, somehow thinking
> I never had a perfectly ideal time in my life.**

The biggest price to living life this way is that I gave up so many opportunities while trying to make everything fit into my imagined ideal of nostalgia, I was never able to be present in the moment, or ever find a sense of peace about what is. My divorce felt very much like the pinnacle of this type of thinking. I was convinced the best of my life had already happened. I had destroyed my one true chance at happiness and acceptance when I destroyed my marriage. In therapy, I was beginning to learn this thought process was the perspective I was actively choosing—*and did not have to be reality.*

A marriage, like every human relationship, is composed of two parties. Two people come together and agree they will stand by one another through good times and bad times. I was not the only party in my first marriage who did not stand by his end of the bargain. Both of us, for equally valid reasons, made decisions that were not conducive to a successful marriage. Both of us, I believe, realized we had made a mistake by getting married. If the marriage had not fallen apart because of my mental health and addiction struggles, it would have had one of two other endings. Either we would have continued on forever, even though we were not in it for the right reasons, or we would have dissolved the relationship through some other conflict. Divorce is not always the right choice. Sometimes couples give up because things get too hard, when they could find other ways to work things out, like through therapy together, better communication, etc., etc.

In our case, Mason and I were not right for one another. We thought we were in love and wanted to commit to each other, and perhaps we were. We gave it our best efforts, but how could we ever have rebuilt a functional marriage when it was not initially a good match. I suppose it would have been easier to accept had we broken up as boyfriends rather than as husbands, but in the end, although it did not feel that way at the time, it was the best thing to happen to either of us. My decision to change my perspective on the ending of my first marriage ultimately prepared me for a relationship and marriage that would bring me happiness beyond my greatest dreams.

Chapter 15

Meeting Brian Garland, the Love of My Life

When I went to a Narcotics Anonymous meeting on March 10, 2009, I had no idea that I was about to find a man with whom I would be brave enough to try again. When I introduced myself to Brian that night, I had no intention of anything other than welcoming someone new to the meeting. We talked for a few minutes and seemed to hit it off so we decided to go out the next day for some lunch to get to know each other. We were both in the midst of taking responsibility for our own choices and responsibilities in our prospective lives.

Brian came to Minneapolis a year after I did, and in much the same way as I had. He needed help with alcohol dependence, and, like me, decided to stay in the area after attending inpatient treatment. I had recently reentered the dating arena, and was finding it to be a very different experience than ever before. Instead of trying to make someone into my dream guy, I was instead taking care of my needs first and foremost, and being open to the experiences of an intimate relationship with someone else. To this point, although I had found a few men I was attracted to and enjoyed their company, I had not yet had a connection the likes of one I thought could result in a meaningful romantic relationship.

We decided to have lunch together, but soon both discovered we had a mutual connection and attraction on many different levels. Our enjoyable conversation lasted several hours. After lunch we continued to spend the rest of the day together. We talked about everything with ease and a sense of mutual understanding. We seemed to have enough commonality and differences between us that what was happening, was happening naturally. We continued seeing one another often, and made a life-changing agreement with one another. Brian and I both had a lot of work to do on our own chemical, psychological, spiritual, and emotional health. I was fresh out of my marriage, and thought I would never want to marry again, while Brian was not interested in getting married.

It was during this lunch, while speaking with this beautiful man, in my mind I started to reconsider having a serious relationship again. Brian and I started dating that week, and although we took things slowly, we had already started to fall in love. Brian was newly sober, and I had only a few months of sobriety myself. We both lived in sober housing, and were both heavily involved in 12-step recovery. When we told those around us that we were dating, we were met with hesitation and disapproval from our housemates, sponsors, and just about everyone else we knew in recovery. Nobody seemed to think that we could make it as a couple because we had not both been sober for at least a year. Nonetheless, with honest communication and great effort we did make it.

Just a couple of months into our dating I had a relapse with crack-cocaine. I thought for sure that Brian would walk away from the relationship because of my use. I was shocked when he did not, even though all those people who were against us dating once again urged him to break up with me, and to focus on his own recovery. This is where I could already see how we were becoming a team. Instead of breaking up with me, Brian just gave me the space and time I needed to overcome my relapse, and he was there for me as I did this. He did not judge me for my using, and he did not base his feelings for me on his idea of what sobriety looked like, nor did he base it on what other people thought he should do. He had his own view of me as a person, flawed but lovable, and while there were times that I struggled with my chemical health, he did not let that determine whether or not he could love me.

We decided to date, slowly. We committed to one another to be open-minded to whatever developed between us, but also to be careful of the pitfalls of moving too fast, or trying to be something we were not. We continued to date, and our bond became stronger and stronger. All along the way we kept a few major rules in place. The agreement, which we discussed, and to which we still adhere to this day was this:

- ✓ We agreed that we needed to be strong as individuals, and since we were both in early recovery, we agreed to put our individual recoveries first—which translated into, we had to love ourselves.
- ✓ The second rule was that we love each other. When there were difficult topics to discuss, we tackled them head-on with open and honest communication.
- ✓ The third rule we had was to love others. We did not want to become so wrapped up in ourselves that we forgot what a blessing it was to have valued family and friends, and even find value in loving strangers and people whom we may be resenting.

One day we wrote down this agreement. First, love ourselves. Second, be open to others and God, and love those gifts. Third, love one another.

The cornerstone of our relationship was and has remained communication. Too often people get comfortable in relationships, and then stop really communicating with one another. We are all constantly changing beings with new cells, new ideas, and new discoveries of self and the world around us. Brian and I have tried to really appreciate this fact, and embrace the changes that have come along the way.

In April of 2010, roughly a year after we began dating, Brian and I both felt ready to take the next step. When we moved into an apartment together, we realized that we both were changing our views about marriage. We decided marriage was something we wanted to experience together, so we became engaged. We lived together for two years before we were married in March of 2012. Our wedding took place in Thunder Bay, Ontario, Canada.

Same-sex marriage was still not legal in our home state or the country, and we did not want to wait until it finally was to get married. We ventured up to Canada with a small group of close friends and got married. About five months later we had a larger reception in Minneapolis with family and friends to celebrate our union.

Brian and I are both different personality types, but we also have much in common. We approach the world with a sense of optimism, and still firmly believe in those early rules that we established our relationship on. Family is of utmost importance to us. We want to be actively involved with our families, and have them know us as a family. Brian has had to learn how to live with my mood fluctuations, and he has done an amazing job of not only doing that, but also of helping me to get through the rollercoaster of emotions I often feel. His calming presence and his undying devotion to our little family and our happiness is something that has the power to move mountains. He loves me steadfastly, even when I am struggling to love myself. I can open up to him about anything that I am thinking, feeling or experiencing. He helps me not to blow things out of proportion, and he does not try to take away the feelings I have, but rather he helps me process them so that I can make my own navigations through those feelings.

Our lives continue to grow and change, but at the end of the day, every day in fact, we come home to one another, and there in that time is a sense of peace and serenity that is greater than I have felt from any meeting or any pill. We have worked very hard to make this marriage what it is, and we do not take anything for granted. We are both very satisfied that we did not listen to the naysayers in those early days. We may both have been damaged, but then who isn't. We are still both whole persons as individuals, but we are able to experience most of life together as a team built on love and honesty, even when honesty is hard.

Here is a quick story of how this way of thinking can make so much difference in this world. My mother, whom I simply adore, is not comfortable with my husband, Brian, and me sleeping together at her house. It has nothing to do with love. She loves me in a way I can never even begin to comprehend, and she feels the same about my husband. She is happy we are happy. However, if we stay at their house in the same bed, it feels to her like she is condoning our homosexuality as perfectly acceptable, which is in direct violation of what her belief system means to her. I think this is more than fair, and I respect her feelings, as does my husband. I told my mother I was not willing to sleep in a separate bed or room, as this is my husband, and doing so would feel degrading to our marriage and relationship. She respects my feelings on this, and I respect hers. So, when we did visit, we would stay at a friend's house. During our visits we have the most wonderful time with my family, and nobody is in a position that makes them at all uncomfortable.

Chapter 16

The Two Ends of the Co-dependence Continuum

Brian and I had no idea then that we were building a cornerstone the likes of which was previously unparalleled in our lives. We were both engulfed in the transition of healing. Our souls, hearts, and minds had been damaged by our previous relationship pains, as well as by the addictions that had derailed us. We had many of these conversations in those early months of our relationship. We had wonderful times together, as we laughed with one another, and developed an intimacy based in the most genuine of friendships. Sometimes one of us would feel as if we needed the other, and when this happened, we looked within and deciphered what we were actually feeling.

This sense of codependence had never brought anything good to either of us, so it was quickly apparent *being codependent* was not what we wanted. Needing someone else in order to feel happy is a treacherous slope. In the end we decided those feelings were based in instant gratification, and was not what we wanted from this newly forming relationship. So, when we had to back off and work on our own selves, we did. We kept one another in the loop through honest communication, but ultimately I was responsible for my own happiness, and Brian for his.

Lust and the desire to be completed by a relationship are tricky ideas to navigate because they feel *so much like genuine love*.

Codependence is one end of the pendulum. The other end, a sense of disconnection or just a sense of total independence, may at first seem to be a bad thing, but it isn't. The problem occurs when either of these things are taken to the extreme. Being so independent that you start thinking you can do everything in life without anyone's help can suffocate one of the most beautiful parts of being human: connectedness.

Think of it this way: In the animal kingdom, species birth their young and raise them for different lengths of time. The "raising" is a feature of survival. Teach your young to be able to fend for themselves. Feed and shelter them from harm, then let them go and take care of themselves. Humans raise their young for some twenty years. We feed, clothe, teach, protect, discipline, guide, and elevate our young; the list goes on. Once our offspring are taking care of all these needs on their own, we still have this great desire to maintain a relationship with our children, and them with us. At some point our children don't "need" us anymore, but hopefully there is still some dependence on each other out of choice.

Unlike other species, we humans learn we can change the relationship from *one of need to one of desire*. We have emotional connections with one another the likes of which is unseen in any other species. This is what Brian and I were finding in one another—*a desire* to share everything with one another, but not *a need* to do so. It was a choice. It was and remains to this day, an interdependent relationship. It works only if we are brave enough and wise enough to be self-responsible, and still remain vulnerable with one another.

When Brian and I decided it was the right time to consummate our relationship, we found that in past relationships, we had been using sex for all the wrong reasons. We were both overwhelmed with what we experienced from the completely unifying force of sharing our whole selves with one another in celebration of our desires, our vulnerabilities, and ourselves. To this day, after more than eight years together, we feel this height of connection when we are physically together. I believe "God" is present in every living being. When Brian and I are with one another sexually, I can almost see the face of God. This reclamation of sex in my life was transformative in my multitude of health struggles. I no longer carried any of the lies I had been told by my religion of origin. I am a gay man, whose very DNA attracts me to other men. This is not a sin; it is one expression of an all-loving god.

As a direct result of my relationship with Brian, my shame over being afflicted with bipolar disorder, HIV, and chemical dependence began to at long last subside. He showed me, through his actions of love, that my mental health struggles did not scare him away. He was not interested in abandoning me when things became confusing or difficult for him. As a result I was willing to be completely open with him about my thoughts, my depression and anxiety, my insecurities and irrational thoughts. I accept him as a recovering alcoholic who found his help from the 12-step model of Alcoholics Anonymous, and I accept that he no longer participates in that program. He accepts that I no longer draw my support and strength from 12-step meetings, but rather have found my truth and strength from a harm-reduction model of recovery. The time we spent involved in that program was a huge part in our evolution as people. We both have our own definition of what chemical health means to us, and we respect and embrace it in one another. We both believe there are many ways to find self-satisfaction, and we choose to find this satisfaction as a team.

As far as HIV is concerned, when I was diagnosed I never thought I could ever find a partner who was HIV-negative and was willing to be with me, but Brian is. We are able to maintain a completely healthy and flourishing sex life, and it has gotten better as the years have passed. We decided through education and deep personal communication how to maintain my health as a man with HIV, and how to maintain his health and negative status.

Physically, I am far healthier than I was before I contracted HIV. My doctors are ecstatic with the way my body is improving, not worsening. I take Triumeq®, an antiretroviral medication every day, without fail. I faithfully see my physician every three to six months. I am abundantly aware of how my body works and reacts, and I know when I need any type of medical attention. Fear has no place in my physical life. I own every facet of who I am, and I am so very proud and grateful for whom this person is. Yes, I do have scary times, or struggles with acceptance at times. It is my overall assessment of my situation, and I do the very best I can, which is enough. Brian remains HIV-negative, navigates my mood swings and medical afflictions with ease, and is always supportive and supported. He has his own psychological issues he works through alone and also with me.

Kathy's Notes—March 17, 2009:
I'm not sure Daniel knows how spiritually sound he is in his thoughts about seeing God in Brian and every living thing! God in nature and human beings is theologically astute and the basis of Benedictine spirituality, which I follow. You must be *in* the world, not *of* the world, but *in* the world is indeed where we see God.

Daniel went home to see his family. He said he had a "different kind of energy"—a huge craving for crack that was almost too hard to overcome, but he did. This craving could be stress about visiting family, or could be Daniel's first drug of choice spontaneously popping into his head. Daniel said he and Brian did an "expectations list," which is their own creation based on the idea they had to be realistic about what Daniel might expect from the family visit.

Daniel's mood is stable, but says the next step is HIV meds, since his viral load is still fairly high: 39,000. I asked Daniel what this meant to him, and he said he felt it "supported life." Whew! Maybe we're getting somewhere, as Daniel believes he deserves to live.

April 6, 2009:
Daniel is sluggish, low energy, sleeping a lot, and getting anxious about HIV meds. His infectious disease doctor prescribed Atripla®, but will need to talk to Dr. Grant about side effects when combined with his psychotropic medications.

NOTE: Atripla® is a brand name for a triple drug cocktail used once daily to suppress HIV. Its generic formulary is efavirenz, emtricitabin and tenofovir. It is more commonly known as antiretrovirals and prevents the HIV cells from destroying the immune system cells called T-cells. Main advantage is with combining three dugs in a simple dose, it increases med compliance.

Daniel was infected in March 2008 when a man told him he was going to infect him. When Daniel sero-converted, he was very sick, and that's when he had the experience at a sober house—when he was told he needed to reveal his HIV status to all the residents. At the time Daniel was infected, his attitude was, "Who cares. I'm not worth anything, and I am willing to cross any line." Sad, so sad.

April 9, 2009:

Daniel was using again, got robbed, and the assailants took his car as payment for drugs. He reported this to the police, and the men who robbed him were subsequently arrested. Daniel reports that Atripla is causing him to have "crazy dreams." A friend/acquaintance committed suicide (unfortunately not so rare in these circles), and Daniel said this triggered his use. He decided not to tell his parents.

Each time Daniel uses, we discuss the need to tell his parents—and whether that would help them understand the extent of his addiction. Would it help Daniel? No fixed rule, but telling the parents each time he uses doesn't seem to be in anyone's best interest at this time. We had to discuss the difference between *secrets* and *privacy*—not everything needs to be shared with everyone. The virtue of *discernment* is constantly being addressed and practiced in the art of therapy.

A challenge working with chemically dependent people is that they always have a reason for the use. While this is good information, and needs to be discussed, their thinking needs to change in some way so they have *no* reason to use—other than it's your choice at the moment. Rather than have clients describe themselves as *alcoholic* or *addict*, I prefer the behavior approach, e.g., "When I get stressed out, I drink way too much at times, and this has really caused a lot of problems in my life." That statement implies responsibility for the behavior, acknowledges consequences, and leaves the option of changing that behavior.

April 27, 2009:

Daniel somehow feels the robbery was like being raped, and it brought up thoughts of "Once again I couldn't take care of myself." In the last relapse, he used crack, not meth, and no sex was involved. From a harm-reduction perspective, this was a better choice. Before the robbery took place, Daniel said he felt "usey," but was reluctant to tell anyone. The word *usey* is something I heard a client say many years ago as he was trying to fight off a crack urge. He said, "I felt so usey I had to stay in bed all day." While probably not in any dictionary, I can't think of a better way to describe the urge to use.

Major issue in recovery: you *must* tell someone if you want to use, are using, have used, and if it is the latter, you should tell as soon as possible. If a client is in a 12-step group, and I ask if he has told his group about his slip or urge to use, he will often say no—either because he feels ashamed, or "I don't want to give the newcomer the wrong impression." This is sad, because the person needs the most support and acceptance, because it is part of his dishonesty. A major consequence of Daniel's most recent use is that his dad said he wanted no contact for one year. Fortunately, his mother did not say the same thing.

Kathy's Comments—May 2009

I go to San Francisco once a year, and right before leaving, Daniel laughingly said something about not having to worry about getting any frantic calls from him this time. On Sunday, May 4, my friends and I were having brunch on the patio of a restaurant in San Francisco, when I noticed I had a voice message. It was from Daniel saying he had a serious relapse on meth, had been mugged, robbed, and was gone from home for two days, but was safe back home.

As is his pattern, Daniel told Brian he was going to meet a friend when in fact he was going to find meth. And when he did find meth, he shot up a gram at a time, enough, from what I understand, to be lethal. Of course I called right away, spoke to Brian who answered the phone, and then spoke with Daniel. He sounded okay but said he didn't remember much of what had happened. When he did at last call home, Brian came with two friends to get Daniel from north Minneapolis. Daniel was disheveled, had a black eye, and was wearing no pants. It is a miracle Daniel wasn't hurt more than he was. Daniel said he felt like he was watching someone else while he was in this manic state, for example, when he opened up the sunroof in the car and howled at the moon.

Anecdotally, I have had other clients describe this same dissociative feeling when in a manic state. Daniel had a session the next day, Monday, when I was back in the office. Daniel looked and sounded very good, considering the circumstances. We talked about what, if any, things might have triggered this episode. Daniel had seen a movie where the actors were using crack, and he had admitted in group that this was very hard for him to watch. He is also struggling with the fear of being honest with those he loves about this episode of mania and use. He is scared that he will be judged harshly and punished emotionally for this use, which never helps anything. He said, "I didn't want to admit how hurt I felt because I shouldn't feel this way." (My thoughts: "Damn those 'shoulds'"!) Daniel continued, "I was already past the point of caring what people thought."

We planned for Daniel and Brian to come in on Thursday, but this did not happen. Brian emailed that night saying Daniel had crashed, was either sleeping or was catatonic-like when he would be awake for only a few minutes. The email was poignant: Brian scared to death that every couple of months Daniel will re-enact this self-destructive scenario, and could die the next time…or the next time. Brian concluded, "I am struggling to keep hope, but managing."

I gave Brian the number to Hennepin County Crisis, which has a program called COPE. If called, two mental health professionals will come to the house and do an assessment. I urged Brian to call them to validate that it was a viable option for him if Daniel was in danger of self-harm. Brian did talk to someone from COPE, and even though he did not ask them to come, Daniel was furious, saying he wouldn't be "locked up." I assured Brian that I would take all the blame/responsibility for giving him the crisis number, and told him Daniel was not acting rationally at this time.

The next night, I received several texts from Brian. He was still concerned about Daniel's mood—sleeping a lot and basically non-responsive. My timeline gets a little fuzzy here, but I believe it was Sunday when Daniel texted that he was up and about and feeling better. He had talked to Dr.

Grant who urged Daniel to not let this go on as long next time, specifically, to call him if depression lasts more than two days. Dr. Grant also suggested keeping a "mood journal," which could provide a pattern of mood changes, and be helpful in intervening before either the depression or the mania reaches dangerous levels.

Right now, May 29, Daniel is functioning well on all levels: physical, mental, spiritual, and chemical. I needed some time before writing my feelings about all of this, and concluded that my emotions were sadness, frustration, helplessness, fear, and anger—at him being diagnosed with bipolar disorder, certainly not at Daniel. As horrible as these episodes are, Daniel, Brian and I learn something new each time, which can hopefully provide us with more coping skills if there is a recurrence. Another benefit is that by going through Daniel's mania and depression, it is extremely helpful in dealing with other bipolar clients. I continue to welcome bipolar clients. Almost without exception, they are sensitive, caring, deep, interesting, and certainly *never boring*. Even the brilliant Dr. Grant has said there is so much we don't know about bipolar, but I will never give up hope and trying new things. It is professionally challenging to be creative in my approach, and I firmly believe the rewards far outweigh the challenge of working with men and women who are bipolar.

Daniel's Point of View

If it seems that my struggle with my chemical health and mood fluctuations never stabilizes, it is because of the nature of bipolar disorder. I have many diagnoses, and most of them are controllable with proper medication and lifestyle components. For instance, my diabetes is controlled with two different medications, daily insulin injections, a healthy diet, and exercise. When I am compliant in all these areas, my blood sugar is stable and at a healthy number. If I start overeating or miss taking my insulin, the number becomes unbalanced again.

With the bipolar disorder, we are constantly adjusting and readjusting the medications as the illness symptoms dictate. I am able to better my stability and chances for less fluctuation with some behavior modification. I notice that what and when I eat affects my moods. I also am very sensitive to sleep patterns. Too much sleep, and I can become depressed. Too little, and I can become manic. Of course depression makes me exhausted, and mania makes it almost impossible to sleep.

Some days, because I take some fourteen prescriptions, about thirty-five pills a day at various times, I simply have to spend the day sleeping just so my body can function. As you read through the case notes, you are exactly where I was during this time. *My battle for stability has been never-ending.* I have had to remain ever vigilant of every mood swing, every change in my weight or environments, as well as every action and reaction with other people. *Living with bipolar disorder is not for the weak.* To remain healthy takes constant work. Things seen and unseen can affect my mood so dramatically I can go from feeling happy and content to fighting suicidal thoughts in a matter of minutes.

Over time, and with tremendous self-education about my body, how it works, and what it responds to, has made this constant state of awareness less tedious overall, and almost second nature. This all took perseverance and determination. I consider myself very fortunate. The tremendous amount of support I have had from professionals, my immediate family, and my close friends, have all made it possible for me to learn how to live—not as a slave to my conditions, but rather as a very functional, safe and sane person as I live my own life. I have bad periods when I need to back down into myself and get through things, and sometimes these periods cost me the ability to be as involved as I want to be with everything and everyone. Those times are definitely worth it for me as they help me appreciate the better and more stable times, and have helped me to have a very unique take on life and its components.

Many people are not able to find what works for them before their time runs out. Still countless others turn to addictions of substances and behaviors, alienating them from their friends, families, and the world around them. The "Bipolar Curse," as I call it, is this. I have to be more in touch with my emotional, physical, spiritual, and psychological self than any other person I meet or know. I don't have the luxury of letting something be, or living an unexamined life. It is a great blessing and a great curse all at once.

I know myself and embrace myself. I celebrate who I am. Still sometimes it would be nice to be oblivious, to walk through the day without having to "process" everything.

Chapter 17

The "Bipolar Curse"

The "Bipolar Curse," as I call it, is this: I have to be more in touch with my emotional, physical, spiritual, and psychological self than any other person I meet or know.

The flip side is everyone in my life wants me to be balanced and stable, but often don't realize that they are critiquing every move I make.

If I am too excitable, I am accused of being manic,

If I am overtired, it often correlates as depressed,

If I spend a larger amount of money than normal,

If I vary my routine, then…

I must be ready to be asked if *I am feeling okay.*

People in my life generally either share too much information with me because they think I have no boundaries, or don't share information with me for fear I will not be able to handle what is happening, and I might become depressed or manic. Having a sense of humor I found is the best way to deal with this. I feel blessed I am able to be a confidante to others at such deeply intimate and personal levels.

What a wonderful gift *honesty* is to the whole world. The more I share about my truth, the more honest everyone is around me.

People have told me their deepest secrets because I was willing to share my shadow side. This is my favorite part of how I live my life. I am an open book for the most part, and though some criticize me for this, the benefits of having these connected moments with people who are screaming out to have their own truth be heard, far outweigh the silly fears of "What if someone doesn't like me or what I say." Well, so what. At some point I realized that constantly wanting to be accepted or understood is not the reason why it is important to have a solid sense of self and self-worth. The real reason for this is so that I can experience, learn, and interact with my life and the lives of the world around me in an honest way. I do my best to accept this about other people as well. It is hard sometimes to accept those I vehemently disagree with, but it is not impossible, and lashing out at those people never does any good. The most good happens when I am just present as myself, and accept others on the same terms. This helps me stay stable, healthy and happy, and helps me truly live with bipolar disorder, HIV, etc.

Writing About Being Bipolar

Sitting down to write about my bipolar disorder is probably the most complicated challenge I have ever faced, second only to learning how to live successfully as a person with bipolar disorder. I say this because there are so many different variables and aspects of the disease and how it has affected my everyday life and life as a whole. It can be so overwhelming to even consider finding the right words to help someone understand what this undertaking has been like, but I am doing so, albeit imperfectly. I do so because I truly think the more people who share about life with bipolar disorder and other mental health issues, the more successful those people and society as a whole will be.

The Diagnostic and Statistical Manual of Mental Disorders (DSM) has the following to say about diagnosing bipolar disorder:

Bipolar Episode and Bipolar Disorder

Bipolar disorder is characterized by more than one bipolar episode. There are three types of bipolar disorder:

1. Bipolar 1 disorder, in which the primary symptom presentation is manic, or rapid (daily) cycling episodes of mania and depression.
2. Bipolar 2 disorder, in which the primary symptom presentation is recurrent depression accompanied by hypomanic episodes (a milder state of mania in which the symptoms are not severe enough to cause marked impairment in social or occupational functioning or need for hospitalization, but are sufficient to be observable by others).
3. Cyclothymic Disorder, a chronic state of cycling between hypomanic and depressive episodes that don't reach the diagnostic standard for bipolar disorder (APA, 2000, pp. 388–392).

Manic episodes are characterized by:
- A distinct period of abnormally and persistently elevated, expansive, or irritable mood, lasting at least one week (or any duration if hospitalization is necessary).
- During the period of mood disturbance, three (or more) of the following symptoms have persisted (four if the mood is only irritable) and have been present to a significant degree:
    - Increased self-esteem or grandiosity
    - Decreased need for sleep (e.g., feels rested after only three hours of sleep)
    - More talkative than usual, pressured speech
    - Flight of ideas or subjective experience that thoughts are racing
    - Distractibility (i.e., attention too easily drawn to unimportant or irrelevant external stimuli)
    - Increase in goal-directed activity (either socially, at work or school, or sexually) or psychomotor agitation—both bodily (motor) movement and psychological component
    - Excessive involvement in pleasurable activities that have a high potential for painful consequences (e.g., engaging in unrestrained buying sprees, sexual indiscretions, or foolish business investments) (APA, 2000, p. 362).

Depressive episodes are characterized by symptoms described above for Major Depressive Episode.

· · · · ·

You might be asking yourself, "What the hell do I do with all of this jargon?" I know I did at first. The only reason I included it in this book is that so often people misunderstand the diagnosis because it is misrepresented and misdiagnosed. When I was diagnosed, the doctor did not explain any of what was listed in the DSM. I don't know if health professionals don't do this because they don't have the time, or because they think a patient (without an education in medicine) would not be intelligent enough to use the diagnostic materials to help him understand his own illness better. In my opinion it is a crime to not give more information. I spent years questioning whether or not I even had bipolar disorder because it was never properly explained to me.

This doubt often led to a type of despair that's always the worst, the feeling that *I am, as a whole person, damaged.*

This fear of being damaged led to real damage I would self inflict onto my life in all areas: physical, intellectual, spiritual, and emotional. Whatever the case, I am going to explain it as I understand it. I am not a medical professional, but this is a personal qualification as diagnosed by my psychiatrist. I have had many, many manic episodes over the years, but a few were more severe than others. I'll tell you about those so you can get an idea of the behavior that accompanies mania:

When these episodes hit, it is most profound that I often cannot recognize it as mania.

- In manic mind, to me the actions and behaviors I engage in seem to be normal and obvious.
- I feel grandiose and immortal during these episodes, and thus my behavior is normal and natural to me during those times, even

though when I am not experiencing the mania I think those same actions foolish and lacking sanity.
- I can do anything, be anything, and engage in anything my brain desires.

Unfortunately, the part of my personality that's active during mania is my *shadow side* (explained in next chapter).

Chapter 18

Personality Type to Understand Yourself

First consider the following information about personality types. The following is an explanation of the Myers-Briggs personality assessment as explained by Kathy Vader, L.P. If you want to better understand my point of view and my personal experience it will help to know I am a strong ENFP—Extravert/Intuitive/Feeling/Perceptive.

—Daniel

Kathy Relates Myers-Briggs Type Inventory to Daniel's Life

The Myers-Briggs Type Inventory (MBTI) is also based on Jungian archetypes, and something I use with every client—and especially couples. The original book, written by Isabel Briggs Myers, was titled, *Gifts Differing*. This came as a message from St. Paul to the Romans, 12:4–8: "For as we have many members in one body, and all members have not the same office; so we, being many, are one body...and every one members one of another, having them gifts differing...." When meeting new clients, I often tell them my goal is not to change their behavior, but to understand them because that's the only way I might be of some help. The MBTI is a wonderful way to get to know a person on a deeper level. Myers-Briggs has sixteen personality types, and each one is a gift—an extravert doesn't need to become an introvert; a "feeler" doesn't have to become a "thinker."

So many of my clients have a profound sense of shame, due to their mental illness, their chemical use, or because they are gay.

It's important that my clients accept, embrace, and use their unique gifts in a way that's congruent with their value system, and leads to the fulfillment of their highest potential.

Daniel is an ENFP—Extravert/Intuitive/Feeling/Perceptive

ENFPs are charming, charismatic, flirty, funny, and always ready to talk and play. They are highly intuitive, with creativity and imagination being their dominant functions. Many people are drawn to ENFP personalities, and the ENFPs may have to subdue their ebullient personality so people don't misinterpret their friendliness for a serious attraction. An ENFP is great at initiating projects, but not so good at the follow-through. Being so charismatic enables them to find some willing ISTJ (intuitive, sensing, thinking, judging) to finish what they started.

Daniel's dominant personality trait is his "N"—implying creativity, imagination, and spirituality. He is a person who has no problem seeing possibilities and "reading between the lines." Daniel is at his best when caught in the enthusiasm of a project, and he can easily convince others to see its benefits. You can best describe your dominant personality trait as what you are like when you are *most* yourself. Conversely, just as each personality type has a dominant function, it also has an inferior function, which Karl Jung describes as our "shadow." This is how we feel and behave when we are not ourselves. This inferior function is largely unconscious (meaning we don't exactly bring it on), and it comes out when our conscious energy is depleted—what we would describe as "stressed out."

As an ENFP, Daniel's inferior function is his S (sensing), the opposite of his dominant N—implying creativity, imagination, and spirituality. If Daniel feels disrespected, has his competence doubted, has rules that inhibit his creative process, and is overloaded with details, he could easily slip into his "shadow" S. Since S means sensing, a person with the shadow S can find himself doing something sensing, like eating, drinking, or having sex—to the extreme. They may work harder and longer, but less effectively, having extremes of both emotional and physical activity. One of the great things about the Myers-Briggs are the practical solutions when you find yourself in your inferior function. The ENFPs may need time to stay in their inferior state for a while before working their way out of it. The extraverted ENFP may find that talking to friends will help, as long as the friends don't offer advice or make judgments. Often rest and paying attention to physical needs, like exercise and healthy food, can help restore their emotional equilibrium.

Brian's MBTI is INTP— Introverted-Intuitive-Thinking-Perceiving.

He is intellectual, analytical, and reflective, and loves abstract thinking. Brian is logical in his thinking and has interest in understanding and explaining the world, not controlling it. Brian is just a few courses short of a PhD, and this validates an INTP's interest in higher education and amassing knowledge throughout his life.

"T" or the Thinking function is Brian's dominant trait. He always strives to maintain objectivity and rarely takes constructive criticism personally. Brian's "F" or Feeling, is his inferior function. It is interesting how this has played out in his relationship with Daniel. When Daniel has had meth relapses, Brian has never been judgmental, and only asks for honesty. When Daniel has been suffering from depression, Brian's first impulse was to try to "fix" this in some way, basically wanting to know what he could do to help. The same dynamic occurred when Daniel was manic.

Gradually what Brian learned to do was just be present for Daniel, but not offer suggestions on how he might feel better, calm down, etc. Brian admits this was difficult for him at first, but acknowledged that this gave him an opportunity to use his shadow "F," where he was present and supportive, but not "Mr. Fixit." The differences between Daniel's extraversion and Brian's introversion have not caused any particular conflict in their relationship. Daniel might go out with friends, while Brian may choose to stay home, and each one understands the others needs for being alone or being with friends.

Because Brian and Daniel are both "Ps"—perceivers who tend to prefer doing things in a spontaneous, rather than planned way, there have been financial issues related to procrastination. Facing these issues has been hard for both of them, but it gave them a chance to regroup. Interestingly, Daniel is handling their finances, and is doing this in an organized and responsible way. You might look at this as a way for him to use his "shadow T."

Daniel's Thoughts on Personality Types

Now that you have a better understanding of personality types, it is important to understand this: Just because one person has dominant personality traits does not mean that he always defers to those traits. An introvert can find the need to be extroverted at times, and a "feeling" person is also a "thinking" person. Everyone has *all* of the traits, but uses them in different ways and at different levels of intensity.

> Com-passion = suffering with…to suffer together. Compassion is not sympathy (an imagined transpersonal feeling), and compassion is not pity (an imagined hierarchy). Compassion for others is a basic notion of relating to and experiencing the world with an open heart.

What then is self-compassion? How is it cultivated?

Kathy's Notes
(2010—Selected Notes so Not All Sessions are Listed)

January 8, 2010: Daniel saw his cardiologist whom he felt was arrogant, and Daniel did not feel listened to or respected.

January 21, 2010: Latest increase in lithium does not seem to be effective. Daniel is in distress and I urged him to call Dr. Grant today and he agreed (mercifully, he usually always does!). Approaching nine months of sobriety, which has never happened before. Trying to eat only heart-healthy foods and stick to a 2500-calorie diet to avoid cardio medication, which has unpleasant side effects. Plus, Daniel has no trust in the cardio doctor. Daniel said Brian tries to help Daniel see the "bright side" of things, since he really is a very positive person.

NOTE: If there is one person who knows almost as much about bipolar disorder as Daniel, it has to be Brian. Brian's first impulse was to "fix things" when Daniel was struggling, but he has learned that this just doesn't work. Daniel has figured out what does and does not help, and more than anything he does not want to be treated as a "sick person." This is a very nebulous role to play, but I think Brian and I both continue to learn how to attend to Daniel's needs without "over-pathologizing" him or let Daniel's emotions seriously affect ours.

January 29, 2010: He is angry at himself for being a "burden and DYSFUNCTIONAL." Held his feelings back from Brian at first, but then "let it all out," and Brian stays!

February 4, 2010: ECT starts again. Daniel desperately wants to be seen as a reliable person, and therefore tends to hide his needs from those he loves. Brian has one year of sobriety (from alcohol).

February 18, 2010: Memory starting to be affected by ECT (bi-lateral this time). Daniel sees Dr. Grant today and may end treatments next Friday. It is frightening for him to wake up after the ECT and not know who or where he is. Despite these side effects, Daniel agrees his mood is definitely better.

February 25, 2010: Daniel decided it is the right time for him and Brian to live together. This makes him feel like a "human being." I suggested both he and Brian write down any concerns they have about living together and share them with each other. ECT ended, and Daniel's mood is stable. Daniel went to his favorite AA meeting, but got upset and wanted to walk out. Time to renegotiate? Daniel took a big step by talking to Brian about sexual intimacy—and Brian took an equally big step by just listening and not trying to fix anything.

March 12, 2010: Bipolar symptoms emerge in the form of irrational thoughts of fear of abandonment and profound loneliness late in the day. Has been with Brian for *one year*. Daniel has chronic, low-level worry regarding people judging him for not working. Daniel has to decide whether to continue with Gay Men's Chorus. He experiences uncomfortable social anxiety when rehearsing and performing. We're trying to figure this out and finally decide it's because Daniel only feels comfortable around gay men in recovery.

NOTE: While Daniel's feeling about only being around gay men in recovery makes sense, it is also problematic. I always urge my clients in recovery to make sure a substantial part of their support/social network is comprised of people NOT in recovery. That provides a balance of "normalcy" and is a good antidote against having many or all of your recovery friends relapse.

May 3, 2010: Living in the apartment with Brian "all good," Brian cooks and Daniel cleans.

May 14, 2010: Feels more at home in his own skin, but still "wears a mask" around family at times.

June 17, 2010: HH Program approved, but other than that, Daniel is spiraling downward. He said he is "done with everything, meds, doctors, nurses." We acknowledge that this is bipolar rearing its ugly head, as he is med compliant, but symptoms may have been triggered by the visit home. (HH program is federally funded to help defray the costs of psychological and medical expenses for people living with HIV/AIDS.)

June 26, 2010: Experiencing lots of sexual urges—Gay Pride weekend brings up memories of being raped at Gay Pride in Rhode Island when he was 24. When I asked Daniel what was the *meaning* of Gay Pride, he said, "Rebelling and doing anything you want sexually." Daniel feels a lack of purpose, and feels he "provides nothing for the world."

July 29, 2010: Fighting off exhaustion, but feels mood is more stable and is eating normally.

August 6, 2010: Topamax still working well, but will taper off Seroquel, as one of the side effects is increased appetite. Still a problem, with his triglycerides "through the roof." Will see cardiologist at University of Minnesota in two weeks. Daniel reports feeling exhausted and frustrated, and he's gaining weight because of meds, but afraid to discontinue.

CLINICAL NOTE: Such an ongoing dilemma for people with dual diagnosis of mental Illness and chemical dependence, plus Daniel's third challenge, being HIV+. Medications necessary for one diagnosis cause symptoms that negatively affect another diagnosis. Sometimes people challenged by this understandably give themselves a "med holiday" because their frustration level and/or side effects become unbearable. Wants to stay connected to "core self" and says he has stopped punishing himself for failed marriage, family problems, addiction, and financial issues. I asked how this happened and he said he has redefined success as something not based on professional or financial achievement. Daniel said he is "doing the work by not doing it for ego." Creditors are after him from hospitals, and are calling family members. Again, he says this is not too stressful. This is a "red flag" for me because if Daniel isn't being candid about his feelings about rejection from family—and creditors calling, I wonder: could this be a relapse trigger?

September 30, 2010: Saw Dr. Grant last week who prescribed Chantix because Daniel thought he was smoking too much. Daniel's really depressed and has extreme nightmares where he wakes up screaming. Daniel continues to struggle accepting his emotional illness; accepting only his physical symptoms. His mother and friend coming to visit and will see him perform in a play.

October 14, 2010: He is "down" again after experiencing rage last night. This came after seeing some pictures of himself at 24, in scrubs, was not on meds at that time and felt normal. My thoughts, how poignant and sad! I suggested he take a new picture of him and his 18-month pin at CMA, to celebrate this and make a new photo memory.

November 4, 2010: Daniel says he feels "low, but not in danger." He is very reactive to seasonal and moon changes. His major stressor right now is Social Security hearing January 25. The last evaluation determined he was "too functional." This was a major disappointment and frustration to both of us, and to the attorneys who had been helping Daniel apply. On "good days" Daniel can indeed present himself as someone with great communication skills and intelligence. BUT if one were to review his reams of medical history, there is a huge amount of evidence supporting his lifelong struggle with physical and mental illness. We can only hope the January hearing will result in approval of Social Security benefits.

November 22, 2010: Daniel and Brian's relationship back on an even keel, but many of their friends are struggling. Daniel had doctor visit and was told his kidney function was being affected by some of the medication he is on. Dr. Grant and his infectious disease doctor are working together on this. Daniel is experiencing frequent urination and pain and is always thirsty, and is worried about diabetes.

December 10, 2010: Had a very long appointment with the kidney specialist and Daniel has some kidney failure. Daniel has been on lithium in the past and currently on Tricor for his heart and both of these medications can cause kidney failure. He will discontinue Tricor, and see the heart doctor in January.

December 31, 2010: Daniel and Brian went home for Christmas. Daniel received a new camera and has new family pictures. The biggest stressor was Daniel and Brian having to sleep in separate beds at Daniel's family's home. Daniel respected his mother's wishes this time, but the next time they are in Rhode Island, they will stay somewhere else.

Chapter 19

Extremes of the Bipolar Disorder: Rage and Shame

Both extremes of bipolar disorder can be frightening—to me and to the people I love. With bipolar depression, the fear is over feelings of suicidal thoughts and despair. Hours rapidly turn into days, and the only time spent awake is for an occasional meal, drink, or bathroom visit. Making it through those moments can take all the energy reserves I have for the entire day. It is not a desire to be bedridden, however while in a state of hopelessness and truly bipolar depression, my bed becomes the only place I can be safe. Logic would tell a normal person to get moving, take a shower, throw open the windows, and try to get out of his own mind.

When I am in a logical and stable place, and have lack of motivation or a down day, I do all of these things and more. Eventually I do get away from whatever is bringing me down, and I feel better. While in bipolar depression...I simply cannot. In fact if someone I love tries to help me when I am in this state, I become overwhelmed with rage, and become totally defensive and sometimes even downright mean.

These deep bipolar depressions truly feel like the end of the world is at hand. I have scoured my brain to understand how I have not crossed from passive suicidal thoughts to actually attempting suicide, but as of yet, I have not. I am grateful for this during all times except when in the throes of these depressions. In fact, while most of the time during these depressions is spent sleeping, my awake time is basically spent trying to find the courage to at last put an end to it all, and kill myself. Terrifying? Yes it is, but what's even worse is not openly talking about it in a rational way with others who can accept it as what is without letting their fears of *what could be* overrun the conversation.

In my experience and opinion, this is nothing compared to the horrors of my form of bipolar mania. My mania has changed fairly drastically over the years. In my teens I experienced very little mania. I was not yet diagnosed with anything, and most people did not even realize anything was wrong. I would spend my days in a state of total anxiety and panic. Getting up in the morning was so scary, and most of my nights were spent filled with nightmares.

My anxiety did not come from anywhere rational. I had pretty much the same schedule every day. I would get up, get ready for school, go to school for the day, and return to a night filled with homework. In my freshman year of high school, I was able to push through this and was ranked thirtieth in my class of two hundred eighty by years end. Sometime between then and my sophomore year, things spiraled out of control. I could only accomplish the bare minimum of my schoolwork, doing just enough to get by. I stopped studying for tests, and relied on what I was able to absorb during classroom learning. I would try to study, but would find it impossible to concentrate on or complete tasks. I am a fairly intelligent person, so I was able to get by with a "C" average, even though I put little effort into my studies. I simply did not have the energy to put into school—it was all invested in pushing through the depression, and hiding it from others. Those next three years I went from thriving to graduating near the bottom of my class.

My days were filled with irrational fears, and the nights were spent feeling tormented by anxiety and depression.

The time I should have been investing in the high school experience was spent on the phone with friends, basically trying to get talked down from some edge. I hid this very successfully from my family. Although some teachers noticed that I seemed troubled, overall I put on a pretty good front, especially to my family. I thought they would find out that in my mind, all this anxiety was due to the fact I was gay, and nobody knew, and I was in no hurry to let anyone find out. I'm sure this was a big part of what was going on, but I was also already struggling with the effects of adolescent-onset bipolar disorder, but would go undiagnosed until the age of eighteen. One teacher at the school suspected my turmoil, and without her behind the scenes helping other teachers understand me, I do not think I would have made it through.

I think back on this time, and two major emotions overwhelm me: *shame and rage.* I was so angry at the injustice of my experience as compared to those around me, but kept shoving it down further and further into my subconscious, keeping it out of reach. The problem with rage is although it can be shoved back, it continues to bubble at the surface, waiting for anyone or anything to remove the lid so it can release its steam. It festers and builds, and eventually every perception the angry person has about every experience is discolored by overreaction. I felt the "shame beast" had been growing since the first moment when I realized I was not the same as everyone else—and something was wrong with the difference in me.

There it was, that shame and rage, happening over and over. It happened when I realized I was not like my brother (older by two-and-a-half years), whom I envied, but we struggled to find relatability, so for protection I encouraged him to fight with me, *all the time.* It happened when I realized the others boys and girls did not take life as seriously as I did. I was more sensitive than the other kids my age, and I seemed to be hurt a lot easier. While some kids on the playground would make fun of the other kids, I would internalize the entire experience. I was not made fun of nor did anyone pay attention to me. I wanted to help the kids who were being what today is bullied, but I was not strong enough. Instead I would feel guilty about not being able or courageous enough to help them, and would cry when I was alone as if the bullies had called me the names, or shunned me from the group.

I felt like a hypocrite because I thought if anyone knew my secrets inside, I would be the target. Fear kept me from doing anything in my childhood, but my fear was best served wrapped in a happy-go-lucky outer shell while inside I was terrified that instead of hearing a girl being teased as "Fat Tara" on the playground, I would hear "Faggot Danny." I eventually found my bravery and the courage of my convictions, but it too came at a cost. I turned to Catholicism for acceptance, but did not realize then what I was doing was trying to guilt myself enough to turn straight, and trying to pray hard enough to make the demons go away. I did not know I would eventually come to thank God for making me gay, or that the demons were not real-life ones, but those of mental illness.

What is shame? It is an inner belief that I am not worthy of love, compassion, friendship, benefit of the doubt, trust, and joy.

All of these steps and missteps overwhelmed me with shame. What is shame? Well, I think maybe it is one of those things that differ in appearance from person to person, but the underlying feeling is the same. The list goes on, and I am sure you can figure out the rest. Shame is the shadow side of myself, the dark side, and if discovered, it would deem me unlovable and unworthy of anything positive. It grew to be a whirlpool with a suction so deep it would bring me to do whatever I could to end my life—and be sent to a hell that I envisioned to be total pain all the time.

I didn't realize I was creating my hell through my own beliefs, and with my own mind. I was certainly being punished, but I was the one doing the punishing. I remember that when I finally realized what this was, I also stopped believing that there was a place in the universe called hell. Hell does not make any sense in a mind that believes in God as love. Hell is simply the absence of love. Hell is being so disconnected from one's self that there is no hope. Perhaps souls that live in hell remain there when they die, but I do not think hell is a state of punishment from God, rather a form of self-punishment. I may be wrong about this, but it is just an opinion based on the experience I have had to date. My shame worsened when I became addicted to drugs, when I became HIV-positive, when I ruined my first marriage, and when I had every relapse. The shame only stops when I allow myself to accept that I have a shadow side, and come to terms with it through love and acceptance. This gives me the power of choice, and frees me from the self-built prison. Today it still comes over me, less and less all the time with a lot of conscious change and work, but it is there—and I am frequently challenged to surpass the shame.

Shame happens when I:

- Go several days staring at a blank page while writing this book, wondering why I am not smart enough or motivated enough to get it all down.
- Feel excluded from something I think I should have been involved in.
- Cannot attend a function because of my state of mind.
- Hear a relative who has not seen me for a while tell me I've put on a lot of weight.
- Watch a movie about parents and children coming together in some tragedy, and I sit there thinking I have failed my parents by being gay, bipolar and HIV-positive, never yielding children, never making millions of dollars so I could take care of them, never being the son I have in my mind that they want me to be, even though all of these feelings are not based in any fact.
- Think about people who hurt other people, intentionally or unintentionally, because of fear or lack of understanding.
- To face discrimination based on my sexual orientation.
- See adults bullying other adults. All the old pain, fear, resentment, anger, and shame come surging through the frail glass veneer holding it down.

I don't want shame to happen; however, it does when I least expect it. It does not always make sense. I cannot seem to control it, but I am learning how to feel it and respect it as a feeling, and then put it aside and live, acting and reacting to the world and those in it with the compassion and understanding I am starting to believe *I deserve as well*. I write about all of this in the reflections on depression because that's where the shame seemed to have come from, and because depression then fueled the shame. Every time I have been depressed, no matter how deep or light the depression might be, and no matter whether is passes quickly or drags on for months, shame is front and center. Over the years, I have been able to overcome some of it. In fact, "some" may not be the appropriate word as I have worked through and let go of a significant amount of shame. This is one of the great benefits of having worked with a professional therapist.

The only way to overcome this shame was to walk through it.

I have nothing against cognitive behavioral therapy, affirmations, or any other model of therapeutic work. However, the way Kathy and I have worked has been the only way I have ever found to truly get through what was causing my behavior patterns, and come to a place where I was sincerely ready to let go of the shame, the rage, the self-doubt, and total lack of self-esteem. It might seem a very strange process. If I am feeling shame all the time, why would it be helpful to take a microscope to those bad feelings as a way of therapeutically treating it?

Try to think of it this way. Imagine if you broke a bone, and did not have it set. Maybe it is a small bone, like a finger perhaps. You feel the initial hurt, but then after a couple of hours you realize as long as you don't move it in a certain way, or lift anything heavy, it just throbs. You don't have the time or money to go have it looked at, so you tape it up, and spend the next several weeks keeping it iced, and trying not to strain it. The bone will heal, and eventually you won't have to baby it anymore, but it will keep bothering you a little. It might throb at times, and your strength in the finger will not be quite what it used to be. You will notice you never really get back the dexterity you once had, and soon it might impact the way you function in day-to-day living.

For me and countless others, this is what unaddressed experiences and emotions do. Sure, you can tough it out, and get the basics done. You may even be able to function without realizing you have actual pain underneath everything. You may or may not realize this pain is influencing the way you act and react in your own life. You might even find yourself blindsided one day when you realize that because you never dealt with your own shame or anger and the experiences that caused them, you have overcorrected your behavior in an extreme pendulum shift in the other direction, or you might find you have simply repeated the behavior upon someone else.

That's what the process of therapy has helped and continues to help me achieve. I finally had enough of the broken finger that never healed properly. When I went to see a therapist, Kathy, we had to re-break the finger so we could set it and let it heal properly. I still have pains, healing is happening, and new shame and anger appear, but I am able to address how I act and react to depression and mania, to my various illnesses and their treatments, as well as to myself, my feelings and my shadow side, as well as to others, and to the world as a whole.

A big part of the problem I face is biochemical, so just dealing with the behavioral side of my mind doesn't fix everything. I need to find and stay on the right medications. You may find the right medications for you are holistic, or perhaps you use western medicine. You might find you get what you need psychologically through spirituality or exercise. I happen to believe because of the experience I've had, the more ways we have in our lives to feed our whole selves, mind, heart, body, and soul, the better quality of life we have, and the bigger difference we make in our own world, and to those all around us.

Chapter 20

The Black Hole of Depression

We don't know a lot about the black holes in the universe, except they suck all life and matter into oblivion. Should something come within the pull of these black holes, a force so strong always engulfed it so that it cannot escape. In my universe, similar black holes exist. They appear to be exactly the same as the ones floating around the galaxies; they are not—but they feel like it. The difference is that although they appear to suck all of the life force from my mind and body, *I can* get out of their grip.

The trick is having the right people in your support network who know how to bring some light to the darkness. This network includes my loved ones, my therapist, my psychiatrist, and most of all, patience. In my normal state of mind, I know I can pull out of these most serious bipolar cycles. I call them episodes, because they do come on in the same way as other illness cycles.

Take multiple sclerosis for example. In a person who suffers from this disease, they can have relapsing-remitting episodes. The person may be doing well and feeling good when seemingly out of nowhere they become completely affected with symptoms, like paralysis, tremors, etc. Sometimes these episodes are brought on by added stress or exertion, while other times they can seem to come with no warning signs. The same holds true in these bipolar episodes. Frequently the warning signs of a major depressive episode are preceded by an episode of mania or rapid cycling.

While my bipolar disorder tends to have a constant presence of rapid cycling, the mania or rapid cycling before a major depressive episode will be more extreme and rapid. In October of 2013, I experienced one of these episodes. October and March have typically been my most difficult months for bipolar episodes. I think it is because the seasonal changes, from the summer to fall, and from winter to spring, are the more extreme, and I am greatly affected by these changes.

In any event, this particular episode coincided with the change of seasons into fall, along with some other major changes in my life. After three and a half years at the same address, Brian and I took an opportunity to move into a bigger apartment. Moving is among the highest of stress-related life events. On top of all this, one of my dearest friends moved away, Brian was interviewing for a new job, and we were struggling with finances. With all this stress, the branch snapped, and my mania came on fast and furious.

For several days beforehand, I felt as if I was fighting a low-lying depression; not too severe, but I was feeling very odd. Brian's family was in town visiting, and for some reason, their visit seemed to hold the full-fledged mania at bay, but it took an enormous effort to be functional and active during their visit. Monday afternoon the family left, and Brian went back into work. *Snap!* For three days and nights I balanced a very tight rope of trying to act normal while at the same time, shooting up grams of meth.

While Brian was at home, I did my best to hide the quirks of tweaking behavior. Tweaking is a term used among meth users that describes the behavior they exhibit during meth use. The brain becomes so taxed that people on meth tend to be very fidgety, sweaty, are unable to remain still, and obsess over cleaning or staring out the windows. The behavior is very odd, and once you have seen it personified, you will always be able to recognize it.

Brian knew something was wrong, and he asked me about it. However, in the heat of mania-fueled active addiction, *my normal integrity of total honesty is replaced with my shadow side,* which lies about anything and everything, and will do whatever it takes to hurt myself, and ruin everything I value. This is some sort of self-inflicted punishment, with a seething disdain and desire to destroy everything I value.

When I speak about this shadow side, I do so as if it is a different person altogether. I am not doing this to avoid responsibility for any of my actions while in this state of mind, and that is important to know. I take full responsibility for everything I do in every state of mind, but it is helpful to write about it the way I do in order to show how disconnected it feels when I am acting from the shadow behaviors. This shadow behavior is self-obsessed while being self-disgusted at the same time. It is not the standard picture of selfishness, but it is *just that*. The difference is that I am out to get the punishment that somewhere inside I think I deserve, as opposed to the normal selfish desires of things like money or power, etc.

After spending these days in a fog of self-torture, which is all my drug use ever looks like any more, Brian confronted me. He was no longer willing to feel bad about accusing me, and was ready to shine the light on my darkness. Brian and Kathy had connected with each other after I had skipped an appointment with Kathy. Although both were hurt in some way by my behavior and lies, they reached out to me with an understanding that my actions were fueled by mania. Knowing and understanding this doesn't excuse the damage or remove my responsibility for my behavior. It does, however, make apparent what the first step is to bring me back from my shadow.

Confronting me with reality and truth from a loving and caring place seems to help me start to win back the desire to get stabilized, as well as the realization that I do in fact *have value as a person*.

Within hours of Brian and Kathy collaborating, I was back in a safe place, telling the truth about what was happening, and what I had been doing, and I was in touch with my psychiatrist for necessary medication adjustment to bring an end to the mania. In this instance, we learned that as much as I dislike the medication, I need to have some Seroquel in my daily regimen to hold the mania at bay. Two months earlier my doctor took me off it to see if I could manage without it, so we returned it as part of my pill doses. The immediate effect was not going to be relief. First had to come the depression.

Having a severe depressive episode is normal after a manic episode. The depression was made all that much deeper due to the withdrawal from the meth. Meth causes a surge in all the mood chemicals of the brain. With the meth gone, an even-steeper drop in those chemicals occurs, exasperating the depression. Add to those factors the guilt and shame of my behavior, and you have a perfect storm of black-hole depression. My depression became so deep in this episode I completely stopped talking for two days. My desire for life and living disappeared.

Brian, in his most beautiful way, kept reaching out. He talked to me even though I would not respond. He went about a normal routine of cooking, eating, watching television, etc., even though I would not do any of those things. He let me be where I was at, without either making drama out of it, or ignoring it. After forty-eight hours I started to eat a little, talk a little, and even stepped outside for some air. It took a couple of weeks to stabilize on my medications again, and to find my strength to fight and work at feeling good again.

I needed a few sessions with Kathy to work through the shame and guilt, and find some inner peace. But I did not give up. That's where the choice is, the magical difference between a bipolar black hole—and one in the cosmos. I don't have to give up. I may not be able to avoid mania or depression with only my willpower, but I can decide whether or not to throw in the towel, and let my shadow self overtake all of my actions and behaviors, and destroy me. It takes perseverance and patience, and to have faith that the people who love and care about me will not desert me, and will listen. It takes therapy, willingness to be painfully honest, and even though I don't always feel like I believe in God, it takes prayer and spirituality.

The ironic thing is that my faith is never stronger than during those times when I doubt God's existence. It is the love and understanding of others, along with my own inner strength and inner desire to be and do better that pulls me through. That is God to me. It takes a village, but perhaps this is not unique to someone with mental illness. Maybe we all need the connections of our own villages to sustain, grow, and come through the darkness we all experience sometimes. Have you ever noticed how the brightest times in life often come after surviving the darkest ones? This constantly amazes me, and keeps hope alive for me during the tough times.

Chapter 21

Mania Is More...

Mania is more! Did you read that? I am manic as I write this. You might think most of this book was written during a depressed or manic episode, but in fact I usually write while in a stable state of mind because most of my life is spent in that state of mind. Are you surprised? Most people would be because in my experience, most people think being mentally ill means a constant state of mental illness symptoms. If it surprises you, don't feel bad. Stereotypes are based in nuggets of truth, things that mostly go unspoken. As humans we tend to view the extremes of people and groups as a part of their whole, and make a general assessment, which then gets projected as truth, jokes are made about it, ignorance is filled in with a facade of truth, and suddenly, a stereotype is born. These stereotypes are demonized as racist, sexist, etcetera, but sometimes paying attention to them can be helpful. Admitting that parts of the stereotypes are based in truth is enlightening even if only to understand what you are up against. It also can help to laugh at yourself when you are acting "stereotypical." Of course there is a boundary line—you can never judge someone based on a stereotype of who they are, and things like racism and sexism are horrible and unacceptable.

For mental illness, this is just as true. I have bipolar disorder becomes, "I am bipolar." This thinking leads the individual with the illness to start *becoming the illness* instead of being a person who has incidences of remission and recurrence of the illnesses symptoms. It can influence the sufferer to start obsessing over his symptoms, and thus start exhibiting those symptoms more often and more extremely. The people in his life then start being hypersensitive to the person's actions, habits, tones of voice, reactions, etc.

This perfect storm has become ongoing. The person with the illness is looking for symptoms all the time, and is hyper-vigilant, making *something* out of *nothings*. His family and friends are also under this hypnosis, seeing mania or depression everywhere and in everything. Everyone has their guard up, idiosyncrasies of personality become signs of the illness, and the stereotypes are perpetuated. In my case, my personality is big and boisterous.

Unfortunately my personality traits are often perceived as instability—which is more frustrating than I can put into words. As I said earlier, some people in my life are afraid to ever tell me troubling news because they think it will send me into a depression. Others are trying to damp down my exuberant moods because they are afraid it is the start of mania, when being eccentric and easily excitable is my personality. I know the stereotype because I live it in other people's actions and reactions with me, and because even I sometimes think I am in a depression or a manic episode when in truth, I am simply going through the normal motions of a day in my life.

Because of all of this, I often hide out when depressed or manic so as not to feed any more of the stereotypical fire. I want to treat life as stable and normal, and I want people to treat me as the same. This has worked, but it has stolen a lot from me. Thus I rarely write when in these genuinely manic or depressed moods, both as a defense mechanism, and as a way to be spared the stereotype.

Change is hard, but it must happen, so I am writing today in a manic episode to tell you what it looks like in the most hands-on way possible. *Mania is more…much more.* Yesterday I noticed the mania starting. I was preparing for a dinner party I am having in a couple of days, and instead of going to one store where I could get everything I needed, I turned what could have been a forty-minute trip to the grocery store into a four-hour journey to three different stores. It was not enough to get any type of crushed tomatoes to make my sauce, no, I had to get a specific brand of tomatoes for it to be right. Without this particular brand, it would all be ruined. I also had to price bay leaves at all three stores because $6.49 was too much to pay, and $4.09 was probably not good enough quality. I had to have the $5.29 package of bay leaves because it would be good enough quality without the exorbitant price tag.

Warning Sign 1. While on the epic shopping journey, I encountered what most of us might have encountered. Someone got mad at me for my driving. I accidentally entered a parking lot in what was a poorly marked exit. There was no chance of an accident happening, or me hitting anyone, but someone with a hot temper and obviously quite a few insecurities, decided it was appropriate to scream at me and flip me off. Normally I would not react to such behavior as I think it only brings me to the person's low level. Occasionally I wave to a person who flips me off as I am sarcastic in my humor. Instead, I screamed back, and also returned the same hand gesture.

Warning Sign 2. Because using drugs was how I dealt with and self-regulated manic episodes, I often get cravings for drugs when I am manic. I have learned how to change the behavior through my therapy, both individual and group, and I have a lot of support mechanisms in place to manage cravings. Most people who have had a chemical addiction have cravings. They happen to come usually at the onset of mania, which also happened yesterday. After I got all the groceries put away, I flopped down on the couch to veg out for a while in front of the television. I don't know for how long, but I caught myself after a while obsessing over my veins. I was feeling them, and applying pressure to make them more visible through my skin. I didn't even know I was doing it but I was, and in doing so, my level of craving for meth, a drug I used intravenously, was growing ever higher. When I did notice what I was doing, I stopped and occupied my mind with something else to get past the craving.

No big deal to me, but what if the mania had been more severe. I could have gotten myself into a lot of trouble if I wasn't so aware and so used to dealing with it. Even then, sometimes the best intentions are not strong enough. Now I was starting the *"what if's"* in my mind, a terrible mental space to be in. What if I did just a little? No one would know. What if I just gave up because it is so tiring to be ever mindful of my feelings?

Warning Sign 3. By now, the warning signs had my attention. My irritability level was extremely high. It takes a lot to irritate me normally as I have a high tolerance for most things and people. By the time I picked up the take-out Chinese food we ordered for dinner, I had been simmering for several hours. When I found myself waiting for forty minutes for the take-out order to be finished, I was ready to take off someone's head. I was angry at the woman who cut in line, and kept calling her a fat bitch in my mind. I was angry at the guy who was working his ass off behind the register for not understanding English well enough, and for constantly making me repeat everything. I was angry at the guy who pulled his car too close to mine, causing me to have to wait to pull out of my space after he did.

When I got home, I ate. Oh lord, did I eat. During the past several weeks, I had been exercising every day and eating a diet with very limited processed sugar, and lots of whole foods, but everything in moderation. Chinese food was my cheat for the week. *Mania is more.* I ate four helpings of lo mein, and a huge order of sweet and sour chicken. I was salivating to the smells and taste of the grease and the sauces. I ate a twelve-piece order of cream cheese wantons, all dipped in the sweet/sour sauce. I ate fried rice. I ate and ate, and when I was bursting at the seams, I ate a little more. I ate until it hurt so bad I could hardly move. I spoke with Brian about the symptoms, and took some extra Saphris® before bed.

NOTE: Saphris is a brand name of a medication called asenapine. It is classified as an anti-psychotic medication, and it changes the actins of brain chemicals.

I have instructions from my psychiatrist to take an extra pill when mania symptoms arrive so I can get the episode under control before it controls me, and literally goes out of control. We went to bed, and I hoped for the best, which would mean the episode was tamed by morning. It was not. It was better because it had not become more severe, but it had not completely passed yet.

The next morning, this morning in fact, my husband and I went down to our gym to work out. I got through two sets of weights, and we were trying a new move. I could not get my muscles to do this lift, and instead of being patient and letting Brian explain why I could not make the lift, I threw the weights on the ground. I rushed upstairs and went to bed, pulling the covers over my head. When Brian came in to ask what was wrong, I kept yelling at him to leave me alone. Brian has a pretty good idea after all these years of when he can help me through something, and when he needs to let me be until it passes. This was the latter.

After he went to work, and I slept for the next six hours, with a feeling of being paralyzed. I was too afraid to do anything but sleep. I was angry, sad, scared, frustrated; a whole melting pot of emotions so strong I could not move. After I had waited it out and the feeling passed, I got up late afternoon and did my workout. I wanted to go to McDonalds and binge eat—and a few weeks ago I might have, but since I have made some progress losing weight, and feeling better with less sugar, I stayed home.

I turned instead to my dominant personality attributes, which is sensing. Instead of food, I did the treadmill. Instead of looking for something to end the mania, I decided to write about it. I can feel that this manic episode is almost passed, and I am tired, and my emotions are losing strength. But harm reduction won out in this episode. I over-ate and went through several hours of feeling overwhelmed by emotion, but I also leaned on others, and I kept myself safe, and I wrote this section. I also went from binge eating Chinese food, and hoping for a caloric meltdown, to binge eating grapes and doing my workout. Even in mania I am learning that *I am not powerless*. People don't have to worry about my behavior in mania or depression, I can handle it, and when I cannot, I turn to others for help. I have nothing to fear, except ignorance, and I hope writing this entry helped with that. I also have to constantly accept that I, too, am only human and flawed.

Tomorrow I'll make my meatballs for the dinner party.

Kathy's Notes—2011 (Not All Sessions Are Included)

January 14, 2011: Very tough joint session with Daniel and Brian. Daniel said he was "all over the place, went manic, and totally stopped sleeping." (Oh yes, this IS mania.) Dr. Grant doubled Seroquel, but now he sleeps all day! Brian very concerned about Daniel losing hope, and maybe, ultimately losing Daniel. Daniel cried throughout most of the session, said he is exhausted and trying to hold on to the relationship, although Brian has given him no reason to doubt his commitment.

CLINICAL NOTE: I feel such anger at this illness because bipolar seems to strike the most promising, young, brilliant, sensitive people. I have learned to help Daniel articulate his anger at the diagnosis, which is so justified—but will it help him really accept how much this affects his life?

February 21, 2011: Daniel is very irritable, and people are getting on his nerves. He said he was so depressed over the weekend he had some suicidal thoughts.

NOTE: I think: is this really fair? He barely gets over his mania, and now he's depressed? (Oh, I keep forgetting…he's bipolar!) Daniel has even had thoughts and dreams about leaving Brian, although we are seeing this as part of the depression, not something he really wants to do.

March 30, 2011: Change of season is the worst time. Daniel is experiencing excessive sweating and exhaustion. He feels "unbalanced," and even pulls away from Brian and may be sabotaging this relationship. Daniel says he would like to "disappear and have no responsibility or connection." Somehow he thought things would get better, and they are not. Daniel needs to let Brian, me, or someone he trusts know when he is having suicidal thoughts, but it is very hard for him to share his vulnerability. Daniel realizes he fluctuates between seeking out his mother, and hiding from her. What great insight! Will try to do neither, but just "be there."

April 26, 2011: Still feels a "little down," experiencing dread and anxiety about going to any outside event. Daniel is questioning the amount of Topamax he is taking, and he will discuss this with Dr. Grant. He is losing faith in the medical profession. Daniel said a part of him "misses the freedom of no meds."

NOTE: Okay, could be that taking meds is a daily reminder of being bipolar AND being HIV+. Makes sense.

May 17, 2011: Daniel experiencing severe allergies, which reinforces his frustration with the medical profession. Also discouraged because for some reason his insurance won't pay for Effexor. He says his mood is improving, but almost had a panic attack last night. We realized there was a full moon and this almost always affects Daniel in some way.

June 7, 2011: Will fly home Friday for Mom's birthday. Ordered 60 roses for her. Will play golf with Dad for Father's Day. Daniel says he is gradually feeling better about himself and more comfortable with his family. We discussed "making mistakes vs. bipolar symptoms." Of course this cannot be exactly determined, but the idea is to put some of Daniel's guilt into perspective.

July 15, 2011: Daniel continues to experience extreme sweating, a side effect of the medication and exacerbated by the current heat spell. He experienced some strong meth cravings last Sunday, when Brian was working all night. Daniel admits the thrill/risk of getting away with something was most enticing.

Daniel identifies a pattern of dwelling on what he lacks, sees himself as unintelligent and unattractive, and becomes seriously self-critical. Daniel says he "deals with pain in one part of my body by hurting another." He is obsessed with whether or not to try and work next year? Or sooner? Will he be judged by what he decides to do?

August 10, 2011: No show. Daniel called later to say he decided to stop his medication. Although I know this is common occurrence with bipolar clients, it is still scary. This has never worked out well for Daniel, and he agrees when he starts thinking clearly.

August 25, 2011: Daniel is experiencing a lot of guilt and shame about getting off lithium, and how this did not work out well.

December 1, 2011: Recovering from pneumonia, which he gets every year. Before getting sick, had a real dip/depression. Saw schizophrenic movie and he related this to his bipolar. Anxiety level really high. Called Dr. Grant who prescribed Klonopin, but Daniel didn't take it because "taking it meant defeat."

December 15, 2011: Daniel says he is not taking his meds, even though in a depressed state. He is avoiding interaction with others and missed Dr. Grant's appointment. What other things could he do?

Married since 2012, Daniel had given Kathy written permission to talk to Brian whenever the need arose.

Kathy's Notes—2012 (Not All Sessions Are Included)
Daniel was a no-show for January and February appointments, but he sent a text saying he was okay.

February 7, 2012: Will have marriage ceremony here in August with actual commitment in Canada. Very irritated with family, especially Mom, who says she can't come to the ceremony.
NOTE: Encouraged Daniel to express his anger here because he felt he had to be the "peacekeeper" in the family, and has repressed a lot of anger as a result. Says he wants to get a job so he won't be dependent on family for money. Hmmmm!

February 15, 2012: Some normal fears regarding if the marriage will work, which is understandable considering Daniel's first commitment.

March 7, 2012: Came to the realization that he may not have been in love with Mason. He could have created the scenario that since Mason was transgender, he was therefore a woman, and acceptable to Mom!
NOTE: Daniel in a very "up" mood, making me wonder if that means hypomanic, but knowing Daniel, I decide it's not. Allowing himself to have feelings: angry at the drugs, heartbroken, feeling powerless to help sponsee James. Question about part-time work comes up again. Needs to talk to his counselor to see how/if this would affect his income from disability.

Will leave on March 14 for Canada to hold their commitment ceremony. His friend Kate is coming, plus five friends. Mom will send some extra money.

March 8, 2012: Session with Brian and Daniel. Asked them to tell the story of how they first met and what drew them to each other. Very sweet story and I asked them to remember this when challenges came up in their marriage. People criticized their dating in the beginning because both in early recovery, but they continued and developed their friendship into a loving relationship in a very slow, steady way. I feel good about these two!

March 27, 2013: Seven people were in Thunder Bay for their ceremony. Says he feels peaceful and comfortable, and decided to put off work for a while. Dad is in Minneapolis and came for dinner last night.

April 17, 2012: Daniel says he is "settling in" to the apartment and to married life. He will handle finances and try to put $200–$300 month into savings. Today Daniel will have been sober from meth for three years! Will tell his story at a meeting, and this time will make and use notes, including the process that brought him to sobriety. Realized ECT helped with his depression, since he has not been on a mood stabilizer since December.

May 8, 2012: Just turned 32. His HIV doctor re-ran tests and his viral load, T-cells, and liver and kidney function all very good right now. Trying to live as a "healthy and spiritually fit man," and realizes that some diet and exercise, plus the prescription fish oil must be helping. Really likes being a "homemaker." Wants to write, but "can't"—just sits in front of the blank screen. Encouraged Daniel to write just for himself, not necessarily to share with anyone else. This may help to understand and put to rest some of his past demons, such as guilt over gay behavior. Daniel said his shame started at age 10 when he kissed a boy.

June 5, 2012: Daniel related a nightmare he had about not graduating from high school. In reality, he graduated, but there was lots of shame involved in this.
NOTE: These are my observation about joint sessions: With very few ex-

ceptions (one being the session we had before Brian and Daniel got married), these times are very difficult for all of us. Daniel can be withdrawn, petulant, angry, and verbally combative. Eventually, he will start listening to us and come to a more rational place.

Brian listens, but when he speaks it is with the utmost combination of honesty and compassion. I know Daniel well enough that I can take risks and say, "Daniel, quit saying that. You know that's not true." Daniel admits that when he is in his angry state, he is trying to push us away. When Brian and I remind him that it is our decision, not his, whether we choose to stay connected to him, he will usually accept that. The session invariably ends on a positive note, but honestly, I never believe that can happen in the beginning of one of these joint meetings.

June 28, 2012: Daniel tried to inject very large amounts of meth (7.8 grams) over a twelve-hour period—at one time, trying to inject into his jugular vein. Dr. Grant prescribed doubling the amount of Seroquel for at least one week. Again, this self-destructive drug use is how Daniel's mania manifests itself. We have learned that preceding a manic episode in the past, Daniel has experienced sleeplessness. Daniel is still adamant about Brian not taking control of his mental health. This is Gay Pride weekend and always traumatic for Daniel, since it was during Pride week that he got raped. We should keep this in mind for next year.

July 5, 2012: Daniel has always celebrated his "clean time," but now feels this puts too much pressure on him.
NOTE: I have found that "counting days" can be a set-up for many people in recovery. Once a year, or some arbitrary period of time has passed, the person often feels the need to "test the water just one more time." Not necessarily true for everyone, but… This also creates a hierarchy in meetings when sobriety dates are celebrated with those with the most sobriety on the highest rung of the sober ladder, and conversely, others are "less than." Daniel continues to fluctuate in his acceptance of his bipolar diagnosis and also other people's perception of this.

Chapter 22

The 12-Step Recovery Program: Daniel's Point of View

For the first several years when I was involved with Alcoholic Anonymous' 12-step recovery, I accepted many things without question. I had so much guilt and shame to work through, plus understanding that most of the people in my life thought I was supposed to be doing exactly as I was told, relative to abstaining from using drugs. It made me feel as if I did not have the right or the need to question the way things were. I don't think this was a mistake, and I have no regrets about having done this, but eventually I found myself healing from the shame, and evolving to a place where too many aspects of the 12-step model simply did not make sense to me. I began exploring the nagging questions relative to what I was professing to believe.

It all started when I realized I did not believe in the first step of the 12-step program. In 12-step recovery they have the expression: "work the steps." This means each participant should seek out someone else who is active in this type of recovery to be a sponsor, and meet with this person, usually on a weekly basis, to actively talk and write about what each step means. After each of the twelve steps is completed and reviewed with one's sponsor, the participant is then encouraged to volunteer to be a sponsor to others. No training is offered for this role, but rather it's the perpetual sharing of one's experience with others.

It is important to understand that I support all paths to finding one's own contentment and enlightenment. I am not writing this as an attack of the twelve steps, rather I am explaining my experience with these steps. This is so you, the reader, might understand why after five years of participating in 12-step recovery, I decided to discontinue my activity in this model—and become involved in the harm-reduction model. I have already explained why 12-step recovery worked for a long time, and I will further discuss why the harm-reduction model works at this time.

Ultimately every person has to fill their life with a balance of beliefs and activities that support and stimulate their own value system and personal beliefs. In my opinion, it's very healthy to utilize whatever means—from support groups to religious or spiritual practices, to being involved with friends and hobbies, and so on—to create a balanced and valued life overall. I completely support the people who find one of these forms of support to be sufficient, and stick with it permanently. In my experience, after several years, the 12-step model was no longer fulfilling to my overall health, and thus I branched out to include other forms of support in my life, and found my personal beliefs fit in much more strongly with the harm-reduction theory of recovery.

Following is the list of the twelve steps from the Alcoholics Anonymous book, *Twelve Steps and Twelve Traditions*, along with the pros and cons as I thought about and experienced them during my time of actively participating in the program. The steps remain the same in each presentation of 12-step recovery, replacing only the addiction behavior on which the group focused (i.e., Narcotics Anonymous, Sex Addicts Anonymous, Gamblers Anonymous, etc.).

Step One: *We admitted we were powerless over alcohol (or drugs, sex, behaviors, gambling, etc.) and that our life was unmanageable.*
Accepting and professing belief in the concept of powerlessness was very comforting at first. It allowed me to comprehend how I could have done many of the things I did when I was actively using drugs—stealing, lying, infidelity, narcissism, a complete disregard for my safety or the safety of

others, and generally treating my life and the people in it with disrespect. These behaviors and decisions may have been out of my ideal value system, but they were not, in fact, passive decisions.

I may not have intended to hurt people and lie to them, but I did it anyway. After a long period of time passed, and I was no longer facing the tensions of this behavior, or engaging in this behavior, I started to realize *I was never really powerless* over my behaviors or my decision to use or not use drugs. I later came to recognize it was the shadow side of my personality coming out and being acted upon. Free will enables us to access our shadow side of being human. I had to ultimately accept I had the capacity to do things that are not a part of my value system, or that were outright immoral, in order to understand and accept the wholeness of myself as a person.

The more I understood I had the capacity to hurt people and myself, the more I began to accept and understand I also had the capacity to help others and myself. I started to understand, for instance, that I was able to be truly generous as I understood and accepted I also had the ability to be restrictive in sharing my talents, time, money, etc. I may have felt compelled to make the decisions I did by a sense that I had to have the drugs. The power of a drug craving is stronger than I can put into words, and during those cravings, I always found that my ability to make healthy or rational decision was almost completely lacking.

These balancing choices exist in every-day decisions, and are where I believe our free will lies. Understanding and accepting that each of us has the capacity to behave on either side of the spectrum lead to me to fully accept myself as a whole person, both human and divine at the same time. It was easy to call my life unmanageable, but in truth, it was not. I was making choices, and those choices were creating the life I was living. I could have decided to keep managing as a drug user, and existed in a state of making harmful decisions. Had I, my life would look very different today, and I would be living with many more unpleasant consequences. I don't think I would have liked it very much, and it is very possible I could have found myself all alone or I had died young, but it was my choice. I was in fact in need of help, and I don't believe that I would have found my way out of any using period without the help of others in my support network.

For me it was the changing—the not using drug—that seemed most unmanageable. I was good at being an addict. However, I was completely unable to manage being chemically healthy, sober, at peace. So, while I wholly disagree with the sentiment of powerlessness, I do agree with the unmanageability of being chemically dependent. The biggest dilemma I had in accepting this first step as a reality was the choice to start accepting I had free will and a capacity to choose the life I wanted to create by the decisions I made. I had been actively using drugs, stealing, sleeping around, and engaging in a slew of other behaviors common to when I am abusing chemicals, but I have always made a decision to stop at some point. Even people who are confronted with interventions have a choice.

Often these people seek help because they are tired of living in a certain way, or because they are threatened with others no longer being tolerant of the behaviors, but they have a choice—and where choice exists, *there is empowerment, not powerlessness*. Empowerment itself is defined as the authority or power to do something. In this context it is the decision of how to behave, and what values to live one's life by. It is the cornerstone to one's own integrity, so to take it away and surrender as powerless at any step in the process seems to me like a great tragedy.

This point is what ultimately led me to stop thinking of myself as an addict, or supporting the theory that addiction is a disease with no cure. I think there are many cures, but they are not readily available or improved upon enough in our society. We need to find better ways to help those who struggle with addictive and damaging behaviors, medical and otherwise. There certainly are addictive substances and behaviors that are more powerful than others, and some require so much assistance and self-assessment many people cannot or will not stop using or acting in this way. Others find they get what they need from 12-step answers to these questions, and it gives them all they need to move forward in their lives.

I don't blame anyone who struggles to stop behaving in a way he doesn't want to, or is unhealthy for him, but I do think each person is required to take responsibility for the decisions he makes even during the active use of chemicals or other so-called addictions. I don't think it benefits anyone to simply give up his or her ability in order to be empowered, and accept that addiction is a disease that can never be cured. If I agree with the statement that after the first hit of meth or crack or the first drink, I am powerless to stop, well then I am just that, but I do not have to be. I am what I say I am, which is why I stopped saying over and over, "I am an addict."

This is where harm reduction gave me a great opportunity. Instead of trying to understand my behaviors on or around using drugs as a part of an incurable disease, I began to understand the ability I had to create and choose what my value and belief system would be. I was able to look at old beliefs that I was trying to force myself to accept for whatever reason, and make the decision to shed these beliefs, and replace them with ones most sensible to me.

Some of my core beliefs are sort of a line in the sand I will not cross because these behaviors are completely contrary to who I am, and what I stand for. I choose not to engage in these behaviors, while understanding I have the capacity to engage in them if I so choose. Whatever decision I choose to make will bring me a set of results. I know when I choose to behave in accordance with my own value system, I achieve results I can stand by with my whole self. When I make decisions going against my value system, I am inviting results I don't like or believe in, and I find it almost impossible to live with those results.

Step Two: *We came to believe that a power greater than ourselves could restore us to sanity.*

Step Three: *Made a decision to turn our will and our life over to the care of God, as we understood God.*

Steps Two and Three were very powerful for me. At first they were the hardest of all the steps to even consider because I was so angry with God, or even the concept of God. As time passed, and I developed my own belief in who or what God is to me, this concept allowed me to accept that we are all subject to a great unknown in life. Sometimes challenging situations happen to everyone—could be a disease, a tragedy, loss of something or someone important, and the list goes on.

On the other hand, sometimes we find ourselves experiencing things that are out of our control, both good and bad. These things could be receiving an unexpected bonus, chance meeting of a person who becomes a spouse or friend, experiencing the loss of a job or a loved one, or learning something about ourselves we never thought we'd ever have the opportunity to explore.

In my case, it boiled down to this. Things will happen in the world, and in every person's life, which are unexpected and unsolicited. Some of these things will be positive, and some will be negative. The one thing that has held true for me through every one of these experiences and all the other unplanned events in my life is that I have an opportunity to learn and grow because of events not under my control. Some people crave change, and others rail against it. Again, just like in every other area of my mind and my life, I have learned that when I can find a balance between the two, I am able to successfully navigate good and bad changes in my life. I used to drive myself to the point of madness trying to figure out and understand what were the forces behind these events. I could not accept that I was not in complete control, and yet I could not accept that all events were simply coincidence. The second step helped me to reopen the case for a God of my own understanding who empowered me in this life to make decisions, and then evolve from the results of those decisions.

After a lot, and I mean *lots* of work, I finally came to accept that the God I believe in is not controlling my life, offering me good and bad things as he sees fit based on how good or bad I am. Rather, God for me is the understanding I so long for. Some understanding I will receive in this life through my relationship with my experiences, and some I will have to wait to understand until I am no longer limited by my human form and limitations. I do not believe that all things happen for a reason, but I do believe that we can find reason in anything in the form of how these experiences make us grow, explore ourselves in new and deeper ways, and connect more strongly with the expression of God that we all are. In that I find my solace, even when I cannot comprehend accepting what life has presented me with.

As a human being, I make decisions every day. Sometimes my decisions bring insanity to my life, or things I am uncomfortable with, or dislike. At other times I make decisions that bring blessings into my life. The good and the bad are present, and I cannot always control what comes my way. All I can do is live life, and make decisions based on who I truly am, and what I truly believe in, and work with whatever the results are to the best of my ability.

So much in this world I don't have the capacity to understand, but the point of the third step is I am here to try, and ultimately to accept life on its own terms. I find this easier to do when I act and react based on my value system. I try to do what I perceive to be the right thing, and when I don't, I take responsibility for it, learn the lesson, and move on. The best I have been able to achieve is a belief that we are all connected. What we do and say to one another has an effect. God knows my limits in all its current forms. This God is able to help me achieve the concept of doing to others as I would have them do to me in this life, and I have learned to treat myself with the same respect by connecting my mind and soul to this same God.

I believe this life to be a classroom for the life I came from, and will ultimately return to, and I am content to learn as much as I can as this person, even if I cannot fully understand that which is divine. I do not see life as really beginning or ending, but rather just a series of transitions of energy forms. The rest is faith, and it's a gift I am fortunate to have received throughout this process of self-discovery. Not everyone has faith in God, and I don't think understanding God is the important part. Rather, accepting that life is not about only oneself seems to me to be the greater point. How each person comes to an understanding is as different as the number of cells living, which is a truly awesome thing.

If there is one God, "that God" has chosen to express life in billions of different forms. For me it is enough to feel God's presence when I truly connect with other forms of life. Be it other people, my dog, nature, beauty, or awe, it is all a way to be more deeply connected with life itself. I find God in the love and life that surrounds me, and that brings me peace. I also greatly enjoy hearing other people's interpretation of God as it always enhances my own.

Step Four: *Made a searching and fearless moral inventory of ourselves.*

Step Five: *Admitted to God, ourselves, and another human being the exact nature of our wrongs.*

I think the heart of these two steps is well intentioned. Step Four can be boiled down to basically what I discussed earlier about discovering and building one's own value system. We all develop different value systems based on our own upbringing and experiences. This is a wonderful and necessary part of maturation, but at some point in every person's life, it is important to look at the values bestowed upon us from our families, religions, nations, and cultures, and make an assessment of these values as to whether they make sense to us.

Just because we have continually been told that something is right or wrong doesn't mean it should always be treated as such by us. If we never assess and discover who we really are, what we really think, and what is important to the way we exist, we can never claim ownership of our own lives. Some people are born Christian, but they might find more contentment and meaning in the Buddhist tradition. Some people are raised to believe they are capitalists, but could discover they think socialism is more effective for them. The list is endless, and it is of dire importance.

This fourth step encourages people to discover what they value by making a list of their own moral teachings and behaviors. This to me is very healthy. The concept of the fourth step is basically what I have already discussed in regards to building one's own value system. The method this step uses is listing all of the fears and resentments regarding our behaviors, circumstances, and those of the people in our lives, and the world as a whole. Most commonly a list, or inventory, is made of angers, fears, resentments, and sexual conduct. Although making this list, and sharing its contents with someone who you trust, can be a very helpful way to get in touch with your own value system, too often the focus of this step is on the negative choices and behaviors causing harm. While I think being aware of all the bad choices one has made helps the person decide if he wants to make different choices, too often this list is solely focused on the sins of the past, and does not include the positive choices made at the same time.

Seeing both the good and bad choices in the same areas of reflection provides a much more balanced picture of the whole person, and I think would greatly help in deciding what changes the person wants to make moving forward. Very few active and former addicts are not aware of the terrible decisions they made and the hurtful things they did. Understanding when and why those choices were made is better enhanced and understood when the entire person is explored, and sometimes this fourth step just becomes a list of sins as opposed to a manifest of choices.

Seeing that there was always an option when choices were made will make those choices more clear in the future, and will also help the recovering person realize that he is capable of good and bad choices. The effect that drugs have on choice is monumental. The pull of active addiction is so very strong, but even at its strongest, there is still choice. To build a new set of values based solely on what is wrong with you doesn't provide an overall understanding of who you are as a person, and what you value as being healthy. This step touches greatly on the ego, and assumes that anyone who is addicted to something is acting from an over-exaggerated sense of self-importance and obsession with one's own ego.

> **While sponsorship is often a very beneficial tool, a sponsor all too frequently begins to act as a judge as to what is appropriate and inappropriate, what is ego, and what are values.**

At the time when I embarked on this particular step of having a sponsor, I was extremely vulnerable, and found myself, as many people do, trying to come up with the acceptable answers, rather than the right answers that were based on what I believed my life's purpose was. Sharing this list openly does take some of the power away from the fears and resentments there.

I was very grateful to be doing this while also working with Kathy because she most certainly helped me to make up my own mind and opinions on what was healthy, and what was not. By Kathy's observing what I had to say, and helping me to understand that what I chose was a means of bringing me something I thought I needed or wanted, I was able to sort out what I in fact did need, and weed out what I did not. This therapy helped me to balance my ego in a healthy manner, decide what I valued, and what behaviors I viewed as appropriate or inappropriate, and to better understand I was not making the same choices, and expecting different results, but rather I was making the choices because I was comfortable with the results I was getting, whether they were positive or negative. Some people are able to obtain this by working with a sponsor and following the standard set by the 12-step program. This is wonderful, but for me this was not the case, and my fourth and fifth step only set me up for catastrophe in the sixth step.

Step Six: *We were entirely ready to have God remove all these defects of character.*

This is one of the steps that changes a lot, depending on the way it is interpreted. In fact, it is one of the best examples of how the 12-step recovery plan could use some updating. These steps were originally a set of six, later revised to be twelve. When these steps were created in the 1930s, society itself was in a very different place, so much of the 12-step material could use readdressing in terms that would be better understood and interpreted in today's culture. Some people take this step to be literal. This interpretation would mean all of the harmful and unhealthy choices and behaviors people made while actively using chemicals were defects of character, or flaws in the whole person.

I feel this is a very destructive concept, because having someone understand himself as defective is very hopeless.

The 12-Step Recovery Program: Daniel's Point of View

I suppose the answer to Step Six is supposed to be that somehow belief in God and willful prayer, along with active behavior modifications, is enough to free oneself of these behaviors and unhealthy choices. I completely disagree. It goes back to the understanding that the human condition is in itself a state of free will. People can choose whether to believe in God, and neither decision changes the fact that every person has the capacity to make healthy or unhealthy choices, good or bad, that contribute to the betterment of themselves and others, or the destruction of self and others. These decisions and behaviors are not defects of anyone's character, but rather the shadow side of their personality in some cases, and in others, the complete free will to behave according to one's own value system, and to be free to determine that value system for one's self.

This step, as I experienced it in my five years of active participation in 12-step recovery, was too often used as a means to portray people who could not maintain constant abstinence *as defective and unwilling to be obedient, or not strong enough.*

This was absolutely devastating to me. I was all too frequently referred to as unwilling, and "not one of the winners." The shame associated with this was exceeded only by the humiliation of being referred to as a "chronic relapser." It was inferred to me at many meetings that if I only tried harder I could overcome these "defects," when in actuality the defects are part of our humanity. How could it possibly be a healthy thing to deny parts of myself that make me human, even if acting on these things are not healthy or productive? I am not saying it is healthy to keep making destructive choices, but it was only when I was able to embrace the capacity I had for both good and bad decisions that I was also able to embrace my ability to choose what way I wanted to behave. Furthermore, this step is one where many people who are agnostic or atheist become completely disenfranchised with the program designed to be helping them with their humanity by giving power to a divinity that they may not believe in, or that may be just a reflection of someone else's viewpoint of God and life.

This absence of sound psychology in the steps is too often compensated by the word "God" or "Higher Power," and explained by taking the disease concept of addiction to another realm called *spiritual malady*. Not everyone looks at this step or any of the steps in the same way, and for some, this step has been a lifeline to making healthier choices. I am not attacking it, rather, I am sharing the flaw in the wording of this step as well as in the way it is often interpreted onto others, which was very destructive for me, and has been for many others.

Step Seven: *Humbly asked Him to remove our shortcomings.*
This step illustrates, in one sentence, my point about a psychological issue of abusing chemicals or behaviors, and turning what we choose to do into *a spiritual disease*. The only way in my opinion to change a behavior is by understanding why we choose to act in a certain way. What are the rewards and benefits of using chemicals? These benefits may very well be termed consequences because they are referring to the same thing. I used drugs when things were going great in my life because I was scared of success and happiness—and did not think I deserved either.

At the same time I understood myself as a great drug addict. I was good at lying, stealing, cheating, prostituting myself, and all out destroying myself and others around me. In doing so, I benefitted by feeling worthless. This was my consequence, and my reward. That changed when I actively built my own personal value system, and gained self-confidence through trial and error of decisions within and outside of this value system. This did not happen until I embraced my "shortcomings" as a part of my whole self, and learned that I was empowered to act or not act in such a way.

After some time, I stopped looking to destroy myself, and became fully conscious of the fact I deserved something different, and it's better for me. These "shortcomings" were never removed, and are there, and I still can act on them, but I choose not to because I understand more about my values, and the reasons why I choose to act as I do. A wonderful side effect of this has been the good things I do in this life. It used to be that I was good and nice in order to get others to accept and love me. Today when I do nice things it comes from my strong sense of connection with others. It comes from a place of genuine love and concern for *others* rather than *myself*. Because of this change in the core of my value system, I am able to understand the true meaning of giving—and that is one of the greatest blessings my life has ever known. In my Catholic upbringing, I often heard the term "one bread, one body." I love this because it is absolutely true of everything in existence. It is all connected.

Step Eight: *Made a list of all persons we had harmed and became willing to make amends to them all.*

Step Nine: *Made direct amends to such people wherever possible, except when to do so would injure them or others.*

I love Steps Eight and Nine, and think the 12-step model hit the nail on the head with these. Imagine if everyone was able to fully understand the ramifications their behavior had on others and the world as a whole. We are all made up of energy, and all the energy that ever has been or ever will be was created at the moment of the big bang billions of years ago. Whether you believe in intelligent design or evolution, this is a scientific fact, and I believe in both intelligent design and evolution. In this way, these steps are the most unifying of them all because they say whenever we bestow an action into this universe, we are following the laws of physics, creating a ripple effect of positive or negative, depending on the nature of our actions.

> **If we all could understand what we have done and why we did it, we could assess and correct ways in which we caused destruction and hurt in the world.**

Those corrections, or amends, could bring about endless positive energy for our own lives, and the lives of others. It is important to understand that *an amends is not an apology,* but rather the willingness to do whatever it takes to make whole something that has been fractured by our behaviors. Offering an amends is not always accepted by whom we have hurt, and sometimes it is not even prudent to make such an offer as it could harm the person all over again. I made amends with my parents by committing to wholly take care of me—and my health. I never made amends to my former in-laws as they made it clear they never wished to hear from me again. I would have felt better offering an amends to them but I had to, and still to this day, remain respectful of the pain I caused, and their right to simply move on with their own lives without my presence in it even briefly. It could be said that my amends to my family was to be more present, while the amends to former relatives was to simply stay out of their lives. This step required me to be willing to comply with both requests.

Step Ten: *Continued to take personal inventory, and when we were wrong, promptly admitted it.*

This step is all about being more conscious. Once a person is educated about something, like his own behaviors and the consequences of those behaviors, he is no longer shielded by ignorance. He has a personal responsibility that says it is no longer all right to travel through the world making unhealthy and harmful decisions with no consideration for how it affects others and the world. This consciousness allows for the mistakes of humanity, and the ability to correct those mistakes as they happen. Doing so in the long run creates a much more peaceful self and planet.

It is not always easy to deal with mistakes, but if dealt with honestly, fairly, and quickly, mistakes become easier to learn from, and can help develop a much more dignified sense of self. This may seem like common sense to many, but after the assault of values that is active addiction, this takes some time to recover. Truly anyone who is more conscious of his behaviors, and the way he leaves a footprint on the world around him, will be benefited with the gift of a more positive world to live in.

Step Eleven: *Sought through prayer and meditation to improve our conscious contact with God as we understood him, praying only for knowledge of his will for us and the power to carry that out.*

Step Twelve: *Having had a spiritual awakening as a result of these steps, we tried to carry this message to addicts, and to practice these principles in all of our affairs.*

As the steps come to a conclusion, they have the final say in defining 12-step recovery as a purely spiritual means of self-help. I support wholeheartedly the people who have found their spirituality through these steps. For those who think their addictive behaviors are a direct result of *a spiritual malady,* I would encourage conscious participation in the meetings and suggestions therein. I certainly have to admit that my years in 12-step recovery helped me grow in a number of ways, spiritual being one of them. This program, while being harmful to me in some ways, was helpful to me in many. It was what I needed at the time.

> **As they say in the rooms of 12-step, I took what I needed.
> I left the rest and focused on a more
> harm-reduction based model of thinking.**

My own reasons for using chemicals to alter my consciousness, and for behaving in ways unhealthy and harmful to me, were not solely spiritually based, but rather as a direct result of my psychiatric illness and my psychological confusion. I had to clean up the wreckage of my life from using drugs in many areas: financial, emotional, psychological, physical, etc. This ultimately led me to do a great deal of research into different methods of help. I needed to find a way to survive while I better understood my brain and behaviors. I have spent many years in therapy with Kathy, while simultaneously being assessed, reassessed, treated and retreated with psychiatric solutions for my bipolar disorder, both through western medicine and holistic medicine. I addressed spiritual problems I had through a journey of spiritual discovery that made sense to me, and by reading and experiencing spiritual practices from all over the world.

Kathy's Notes—Combined From 2013 Sessions

Daniel and Brian met in March of 2009, dated and then lived together for two years before getting married March 2012. Daniel has given Kathy and Brian the right to speak about Daniel's issues, and at times, Brian joins the therapy sessions, especially following a crisis.

January 13, 2013: Daniel says that sharing so much about his life helps alleviate the shame he often feels.

March 14, 2013: Daniel says little things like not getting a good parking spot are "setting him off."

Both Daniel and Brian are reluctant to tell their parents they bought a car because they are both getting financial help from their families. Even when things are going well, Daniel still feels guilty about not working.

March 28, 2013: We talk about the possibility of weekly check-ins with the family, so that both he and they will realize that phone calls don't need to be about a disaster.

Daniel and Brian establish safeguards to maintain open and honest communication to aid in reducing potential harm from choices made while Daniel is in a manic state.

Daniel still struggles with telling people he wants "to use"—which usually starts on the computer looking for drugs. Daniel says the moments of his deepest shame occur when he is on the computer doing this, and it's when he feels most vulnerable. Should he put some type of "warning" note on the computer to help him resist the next temptation?

April 15, 2013: Daniel was super-religious as a very young man, and now he professes anger and resentment toward the Church. This is a complicated issue: Daniel's mother believes that she cannot be a faithful Catholic and accept Daniel's homosexuality. I continue to encourage Daniel to express whatever feelings he has about religion so that ultimately he will find the type of spirituality that will enhance his life. Daniel is spiritual in its finest sense because he truly believes God is present in all humanity. We both agree that *unlearning some things* he has been taught about religion needs to begin.

Daniel talks about his need for balance and validation. The balance part is understandable if you remember what ENFP stands for. Daniel's habit of doing things to please others helps his need for validation, but this where the moderation comes in. I tell Daniel that learning to say "no" is hard, but something that will eventually help him feel better about himself. Also, saying "yes" when you mean "no" will most frequently result in resentments.

August 22, 2013: Every time Daniel feels depressed, the recurring thought is: "I need to get a job." He says that sometimes it is impossible to have hope because "I have wasted so many opportunities." Daniel is not the first and won't be the last person I work with who comes face to face with hopelessness. Sometimes we, as therapists, need to have hope for our clients when they have none.

August 29, 2013: Brian and Daniel come in for joint session. Daniel is in a manic state—he is belligerent and wants to "quit everything and break up." In his mania, Daniel becomes more and more illogical. Daniel stopped taking his prescribed Seroquel, and I strongly suggest that he contact Dr. Grant as soon as the session is over. Breakthrough? Could it be that it is safe for Daniel to direct his anger at the Church because he knows the Church wouldn't leave him? Daniel says if this is true, it may be time to "forgive the Church."

October 8, 2013: Daniel is tearful regarding his perceived failures. He says, "I feel fatally human." He admits his identity is wrapped up in being "strong and compassionate." Daniel views his multiple diagnoses and his humanity as a serious "crack in the ice" (of his identity). When he experiences his imperfections, Daniel's tendency is to overcompensate back to the "nice guy" persona.

October 24, 2013: Daniel's medication regimen is stabilizing, but he says he is in the darkest spot since leaving college at 18. When his thoughts get out of control, he tells himself "the next episode will be worse." We are realizing that Daniel's manic or depressive episodes seem at present to be coming in three-month cycles.

Our dilemma is whether we keep track of these times and try to anticipate the next phase or, will this result in unnecessary stress. Currently, I think Daniel does remember when he experiences a serious mood swing, and it has been beneficial, since the swings are coming less frequently. Ongoing challenge: how can Daniel experience a mood swing without "using"? One consistent pattern is that when Daniel does use, he will tell Brian he is leaving to go help someone who is struggling with cravings or is already using. Understandably, Brian has become very suspicious when Daniel talks about going out on a "helping mission."

October 21, 2013: Daniel will see a nutritionist at the University of Minnesota regarding weight gain and ways to improve his health without more medication. His infectious disease doctor is going on maternity leave, but Daniel's HIV numbers are great. We realize that Daniel is most vulnerable to bipolar symptoms during season changes in March and October. We agree that being vigilant, but not unduly anxious, during these times would make sense. Had a rough spot last week when he was losing faith in the medical profession, and told Brian he was stopping all his meds. Brian's response was, "Okay." Oh Brian, you deserve an Academy Award for such a perfect reply! Daniel continues taking his meds...

November 27, 2013: Daniel reports ten days of emotional stability, and he and Brian are planning a Thanksgiving dinner for several of their friends. He has had wonderful dreams about his maternal great grandmother and realizes that Spirit, for him, is comprised of the energies of the people in his life. After this dream, Daniel felt forgiveness for himself for the first time and says, "What's the point of suffering?" I had to point out that Daniel has done literally years of hard work to come to this point.

December 20, 2013: Daniel smoked meth by himself at his house, but didn't tell Brian before because he thought Brian couldn't stand to hear this. When he did tell Brian, for once Brian actually got very hurt, frustrated, and angry because Daniel didn't tell him before using. Some very important aspects of this incident is that Daniel:

- Did NOT go into an unsafe situation to use (a FIRST),

- Smoked, rather than injected (a much safer method of meth transmission),
- Was not in a manic state, and therefore did not engage in any self-destructive behavior.
- From a harm-reduction perspective, this incident was a definite step in the right direction.
- From a 12-step perspective, Daniel relapsed again and should probably go back to Step One or treatment.

Lesson learned: Tell Brian if you want to use; he CAN handle this!

Chapter 23

What Is the Harm-Reduction Model?

Harm reduction was a lifesaver because it came at a time when I realized mania was causing me to try to self-destruct as second nature, and solely by impulse. It seemed that making healthy choices while manic was becoming almost impossible. The concepts were very helpful—that I could do everything I could to make the least destructive decisions while in this state. Hopefully I could fight through the mania without drug use, but when I could not, I found I had a much more fluid means of dealing with the impulsive behavior, during and after, through the concepts and support of the harm-reduction model. I was fortunate to have Kathy, my weekly harm-reduction group, and a very intelligent and understanding husband—all of whom were actively involved in supporting me as I learned to navigate this new severity of mania—and come up with a way to navigate mania without turning to destructive behavior.

NOTE: Harm reduction is known as a public health policy or a set of policies that believe trying to change a person's behavior by criminalizing it, or refusing tolerance of it, is ineffectual in most cases. In many of these cases, it tends to cause further harmful behavior.

Harm reduction is most commonly associated with illicit drug use and sexual behaviors, but its theory can be applied to all human behavior. By meeting people where they are at in their experience surrounding drugs, sex, or any other potentially abusive or detrimental behavior, elimination of risk can be achieved by reducing that risk, and over time, the person engaging in these behaviors will be able to eventually learn what is *really* behind his behaviors, and make the changes he sees fit in his behaviors and belief systems.

Ask anyone in a 12-step group or a harm-reduction group what they think about the other program, you are sure to get an opinion. Unfortunately the two groups of thought have come to a place where they seem to be pitted against one another. Twelve-step recovery is based on an abstinence-only policy, while harm reductionists believe, although the epitome of harm reduction is not engaging in risky or illegal behaviors, the reality is that it takes most people time to change and build a solid conclusion of their own value systems and self-esteem to make those changes.

Twelve-steppers believe recurring use, or relapse, is avoidable by actively following the advice given in the steps, working with a sponsor, and getting support from meetings and the people in them. Sometimes this does in fact work, which is wonderful.

The problem: the success rate of 12-step recovery is evaluated to be anywhere from five to thirty percent, which leaves a relapse rate of seventy to ninety-five percent. This is a staggering number.

Most troubling, and again this is my opinion, many times someone who relapses is subject to great shame for his recurrence of use—as if he did not do the program correctly or listened to the right people. Furthermore there is this counting of clean time. While achieving different durations of clean and sober time is certainly something to celebrate, if a person has a recurrence of use in his life, no matter the severity, this conceptual clock is reset to the beginning.

I never understood this. A person with a year of sobriety is put back to square one, receiving twenty-four hour coins and they start counting his sobriety all over again. If relapse is a part of so many people's recovery, why are we scoring our sober time like it is a race in a game? In my early days of recovery, I would frequently relapse around clean-time milestones. The pressure of this race always got to me. For some people this is a treasured practice, so I respect it, but I think it disqualifies the lessons learned during a relapse as something other than a part of the recovery process, and is often counterproductive. I had a relapse once after three years of continuous sobriety. The use was brief. Truly, after entering therapy, any time I ever used it was over quickly.

I cannot even remember the details, but I do remember my absolute dread about returning to my normal meeting, feeling as if I had let everyone down, and worried I would once again be tagged as a chronic relapser as I had been in my early 12-step days. Some people, mostly close friends, supported me graciously and worked hard to build me up. For them, I remain forever grateful. Others proceeded to lecture me about how I was working my program wrong, and others advised my partner to put me back in rehab. What I described seems to me to happen too frequently. I chose to stop using within a day of starting the use, but all that seemed to be focused on was the use itself. If we did this with every area of our lives, our mistakes would surely kill us all.

Recovery seems to me to be more important than just lengths of abstinence. Unless you come out of a relapse and go right into a treatment center, or become appropriately involved in the 12-step model, you are considered dangerous and toxic. This thought comes from a place lined with good intentions, but it lacks compassion, understanding, and tolerance. I suppose this is where my own personal and final split came with 12-step recovery.

Good people in 12-step meetings and communities are doing great work for themselves and others, but it seems not much tolerance for mistakes is allowed. There is a veneer of such tolerance, but it was not my experience that it was sincere tolerance. The first time you go to rehab, you learn a lot, however, after this time, it is basically a $30,000 month of "three hots and a cot." It is a good option if you cannot stop the use, but so often people can and do. I think the rhetoric about relapse is frequently the actual cause of use.

So many people are afraid to admit when they are having thoughts and cravings because they don't want to be perceived as weak, or as not working a strong-enough program. People tend to hide the truth, which is the fastest way I know of to relapse. Many times I have been to a meeting where everyone was talking about how wonderful everything is, and what a gift the program is, but then, someone shares how he is fighting cravings and is close to using. Some at the meeting offer help and support, but for the most part, many others are feeling the same way, but were too afraid to share it.

I do think it is a common feature of human nature. We are all leaders of our own lives, but we are also mostly more comfortable when we are not alone in what we are feeling. Having others express similar feelings is part of what is so beautiful about the 12-step model, but the longer I attended I started to see this happening less and less. We should have a celebration of individual ways of recovery that is stronger than the celebration of one modeled way.

There was too much emphasis on this one way—abstinence only—and it made me feel like I did not fit in even during the ninety-nine percent of the time when I was not using. This is something that I do find in the harm-reduction model: a celebration of diverse ideas all leading to a healthier, more whole person. As I said earlier, some AA meetings actually do not allow those struggling with other drugs to participate. They will announce at the beginning of these meetings that if you are not simply an alcoholic, and are a drug user, you should not speak, but listen only.

It says right in the AA literature that alcohol is a drug, so this always dreadfully confused me. Perhaps my issue with big organizations is the hypocrisy I see that then becomes all I seem to focus on. Others who do not have this issue have different experiences, and I wish anyone in any form of trying to better themselves and the world the very best of everything—and my utmost respect.

At the time I wrote this chapter in 2016, I had been involved for two-plus years in a harm-reduction group, meeting weekly. I have struggled with my own chemical health while in this group, usually as a result of being in an unmanaged manic episode, and each time it is very brief, but just as deadly and risky. The times I have had a recurrence of drug use, I applied harm-reduction principles to my benefit.

The group has always welcomed me with understanding, but more powerful has been the concepts of harm reduction. I never come back with any shame; only understanding. I take responsibility for my mistake, and we talk about the reasons why I made the decision to use. Each and every time this has happened, I have learned more about how addiction seduces me, more about how my bipolar disorder and the feelings associated with it have influenced my decisions to use or not.

Yes, addiction exists, but harm reduction as a philosophy, and in its practical expressions that my group has taught me, I know *I am not powerless over addiction*. I always have choice—to use or not use, to give into the cravings, or activate all of my support mechanisms to not use. I am very gratified to be in a place where I am far removed from my last use, and have no desires to use again. I still get cravings, and I am sure I will always ponder using when in a manic episode, but I have developed the skills and structures from the ground up to keep me from using, and they are strong enough for me to feel confident in my ability to navigate any mental state without the crutch of drug use.

I had to go through an awful lot of bad decisions and consequences to learn how to trust myself, my husband, Kathy, group members, others around me in the world, my family…the list is seemingly endless.

I have been lying all my life, trying to cover up who I am because of fear and shame. It took a lot to get to a place where I could trust anyone—*especially myself.*

Harm reduction has been the latest experience and tool given to me, and like my time in the rooms of 12-step recovery, I have learned how to be a better version of myself. I was able to go from chronically relapsing to not relapsing, but I also know if I ever do have a recurrence, it doesn't have to define me. It can simply be a human mistake, I can choose to end the use whenever I want, and I can pay attention to what is out of balance in my life, which might have caused me to turn to risky behavior in the first place.

Kathy's Notes

Several years ago when I was beginning to get disenchanted with the 12-step program, I shared my frustration with a client who had been struggling with meth addiction. He decided to start a group for men who have sex with men (MSM) who use meth, have a desire to change, but have not been successful with traditional AA, Narcotics Anonymous (NA) and Crystal Meth Anonymous (CMA) groups.

He put ads on city buses inviting these men to a support group that would meet weekly at Minnesota AIDS Project. The group was small at first, but then grew and continued for several years until this space was no longer available. The only "rules" for this group were that no one would offer meth to another member who was trying to quit, and disruptive behavior in the group was not appropriate. Aaron (my client) and I found Patt Denning's book, *Over the Influence,* to be extremely helpful. We also attended a national Harm Reduction conference in Austin, Texas, and were blown away by the many ways in which harm reduction was being used by so many people and so many groups.

So, what is Harm Reduction? My own definition is that individual goals are intrinsic to this theory, small changes are encouraged and validated, and relapses/slips do not require you to start over in your process of attaining chemical health. It is *not* "teaching people how to use," but instead attempting to minimize the risks involved in whatever chemical is being used. AA uses the term "rigorous honesty," and I believe that in harm reduction, rigorous honesty means knowing yourself and what choices you will make to achieve chemical health. "Sobriety" or total abstinence is not necessarily the goal, unless the person chooses to make it one.

This kind of honesty is difficult to attain because it is easy to tell yourself that, for example, although you don't do meth, you can drink occasionally. And yes, this may be the case for some people, but others have found that alcohol lowers their defenses just enough to give them "permission" to use meth. Some lifelong alcoholics *may* be able to drink socially after some years of sobriety, while others find that this is just not possible.

People pursuing chemical health through the harm-reduction model are not required to give up all use right away, but to try small changes in their use while simultaneously adding something positive to their lives. Physicians will still treat people who aren't 100 percent compliant with all recommendations, but will work with the patient to make all the changes that are possible. Making small changes builds the foundation for larger changes, and is a continuous process, not a final goal.

I have learned that in the long run, consequences do not work to permanently change behavior. Just as spanking a child stops the behavior in that moment, positive reinforcement is a much-more effective tool. Clients I have worked with have lost families, friends and jobs. They have been arrested, homeless, and experienced other serious consequences, but have continued to use. Only when people can find something in their lives that is more rewarding and pleasurable than the comfort and escape of drugs and alcohol, can permanent changes occur. In his book, *This Is How,* Augusten Burroughs said, "I wanted to write more than I wanted to drink, and I knew if I kept drinking I could not write."

In 12-step groups, people who relapse are often required to begin working the steps all over, starting with Step 1. Sometimes a "24 Hour Chip" is given to the person who admits a relapse. While these practices can be helpful, in harm reduction, a slip is seen as part of the change process. Most people do not walk a straight line from aberrant behavior to total success, but experience "detours" along the way. In the harm-reduction group I facilitate, a relapse or slip is talked about, circumstances leading to the slip are discussed, no blame or recrimination is necessary, and the person who relapsed is encouraged to create some changes that could prevent another use. There is no glorifying, no rescuing, and the goal is to learn something valuable from each slip—and do something different next time. We realize that it takes time and patience to see the benefits of a new, healthy lifestyle, but that the effort is ultimately worth it.

A final aspect of harm reduction (HR) that is significantly different from 12-step groups is that in HR groups, members are not required; in fact they are discouraged, from identifying themselves as addicts or alcoholics. In AA, members will introduce themselves by saying, "Hi, my name is Daniel, and I'm an addict." The difference between identity and behavior is crucial because how one identifies himself is how he behaves. Alcoholics drink alcohol, and drug addicts do drugs. As a therapist, I suggest that an alternate introduction might be, "Hi my name is Daniel. In times of stress and to change my mood, I use meth, which has seriously affected my mental health," or "Hi, my name is Jim. I love being at the bar and socializing with my friends, but my alcohol use has caused some serious consequences in my life." There is no need to change one's identity, but it is necessary to take responsibility for behavior, and to make changes so that harm to self or others does not continue.

Chapter 24

Spirituality and Addiction—
Oh Yeah, and Masturbation

As I have already discussed, throughout my entire life, I have had a relationship with God. For the first twenty years, it was as a Catholic, and I was extremely devout in my teen years. When the initial onset of bipolar symptoms started at about the age of twelve, I threw myself into my faith. I took a very literal approach at the time to how I practiced, and what I chose to believe. Unfortunately, this faith did not work too well, mostly because I was basing it in fear. I was constantly afraid I had done something wrong.

At first I thought my undiagnosed bipolar disorder was an attack of demons on my soul, thrusting my mind into the powers of evil. I thought I must have invited this into my life, and every day I would literally beg God for mercy. Every prayer was an apology for being such a sinner, even though I was a fairly well-behaved teenager. Around the same age I discovered masturbation. Perhaps the euphoria of orgasm was my first addiction, in the sense of how it changed how I felt. For the time when I would masturbate, I would be able to completely disappear into a fantasy, and my reward was ultimately orgasm, which would feel like total euphoria.

Masturbation is a physically pleasing sensation, but it also releases brain chemicals and changes emotion, which is one of the reasons why sex is such an amazing experience, and is so emotionally charged. Although this is a natural part of adolescence and on into adulthood, I would ultimately feel as if I had committed a grave sin, and this feeling would make the rapid cycling of my bipolar cycles dive deeper and deeper past the states of depression into a state of grave despair. At age fifteen, my Catholic school taught that when I would masturbate, I was literally killing the potential for human life. In my religion class, we learned this was a sin the likes of which perhaps only abortion could rival. I would try with as much self-will as I could muster to not masturbate, but it was a release on so many levels, I simply could not control the behavior. What teenaged boy can control such behavior? It is a normal, natural, and healthy part of growing up—but I could not reconcile it with what I understood my faith to be at the time. I was consumed with guilt, but I was harboring a much deeper, darker secret. When I would masturbate *I would think of sex with men*.

I was surely gay, and in my state of mind, this sin would send me straight to eternal hell.

Eventually, my diagnosis of bipolar disorder alleviated some of the weight of this guilt, and allowed me to finally discover it was not demons possessing me that made my mind race and battle me. Medication would help, even if only a little at times, and at eighteen, this left me with undeniable proof bipolar disorder was the cause. At nineteen, I began seeing my very first therapist. As I journeyed through the psychological make up of who I was and what I believed, I would have to come to terms with the fact I was a gay man, and if I was going to have any chance of happiness, I would have to embrace who I was, and accept it as natural and not sinful.

This is likely the straw that ultimately led to my decision to abandon my Catholic faith, and venture out to find my own personal understanding of everything spiritual. For years I battled God on a daily basis. My prayers throughout my twenties and into my early thirties were mostly angry prayers. I would rage against all traditional understandings of God and Spirit, and would find myself absolutely baffled about how any loving God could allow so much suffering in this world; both mine and others. For a few years I gave up on God completely, and even looked into being excommunicated from the Catholic Church. I tried with all my might to hate religion and people who participated in religion. I blamed God for all the bad in the world, while simultaneously denying the existence of God (so much for being an atheist).

Eventually I started working with Kathy, a Catholic. We often had discussions about my relationship with God and religion, and Kathy never pushed her beliefs or faith on me in any way. She understood where I was coming from, and she did not try to change my mind on anything. Rather, she asked questions in order to help me define my own beliefs and faith. She has on many occasions joked with me about how during the hard times, I seem to want to pick a fight with God. She also pointed out that the passion with which I did not want to believe in any higher power, was a great expression of how much I wanted to, or did in fact believe.

Ultimately, and with an extraordinary amount of work and experience on my part, I found myself coming to understand what I actually do believe. Many different factors went into this, from trying different religions to reading ancient wisdom books. I was able to, over time and with constant effort, come to understand what I believe God and the meaning of life to be. I did not recognize that while I was doing it, I was defining my own spiritual health, but I will never forget the space of time when I finally realized that I had in fact come to understand God and what Spirit means to me.

In March of 2014, my cousin Ryan, who had battled lung disease for over twelve years, finally succumbed to his illness and transitioned from this world at the age of thirty-one. Over the course of the week back home, I confronted suffering, loss, forgiveness, and ultimately healing. At his funeral in a Catholic church, I felt the overwhelming need to accept communion. In doing so, the years of anger and resentment slipped away. I was able to recognize that although Catholicism did not work for me, it is a religion of billions of people who find it does aid in their spirituality. I no longer had to hate this or any other form of faith because of the human ways in which it is sometimes run. I was even blessed with a sense of comfort on a spiritual level with my Catholic past, finally being able to admit and accept the many wonderful things that Catholicism had brought into my life. I did not need to believe my validity as a person came from any religion or that God was only available to those who practiced a certain type of religion. I ceased needing to distance myself from God, and now understood *suffering is a key component to free will*. I even accepted certain aspects of Catholicism back into my spirituality. For instance, I pray the rosary as a form of meditation. I also find great strength and peace from communion at Catholic mass, and when I find myself at a mass of any kind, I accept that communion as a gift of faith.

> **God could be available to me if I chose to believe in things like mercy, grace, love, tolerance, forgiveness, respect, and the unique expression of God that's in each and every soul in human form.**

I have always had a deep sense of connection and attraction to the sacred feminine. I love strong women who change the worlds they live in, and the women of the Catholic faith from the Virgin Mary to Mary Magdalene. This is also a big part of the reason why I am so devoutly connected to my own mother. The strength of a mother is absolutely sacred, and in my opinion, one of the strongest and truest forms of love in existence.

I believe I am here to learn as much as I can in this life, and that I might have chosen these experiences before I was even born. I certainly choose how to relate as a soul every day and through every experience. How I choose to engage, act, and react in this life is ultimately how I will learn the lessons I came here to learn, but I am not predestined, I have free will.

This was a major moment of transformation and the way I live my life. I own my life's purpose, even if I cannot totally understand it, or put it into words. The magnitude of losing my cousin when and how I did, helped me piece together so many lessons that had been so long in process. I forgave not only Catholicism, but also people and events I had been holding onto for a long time. When I returned from the week spent grieving for Ryan, I found myself facing another major fear: my own mortality. The week before my cousin died, I had commented at my weekly harm-reduction group that I was scared of him dying because it felt like I would be next. In my mind, I saw us both as having chronic life-threatening illnesses, and so it made my own mortality seem so much more real. After going through the experience of releasing Ryan back to God, I found peace in knowing there is nothing to fear. I hope to live a long life, but I truly understand there is a time for everything, and all I am responsible for is embracing fully what every moment has in store while being a positive force for myself, those I love, and the world as a whole.

I wish with my whole heart that my cousin had not been robbed of the gift of a long life, and I had felt guilty for years that his illness, which was unsolicited, was fatal, while the illness that I had knowingly contracted was managed with medication. I finally let go of that guilt, and replaced it with a commitment to honor his life and mine by living every day and every moment to the fullest.

Kathy's Notes—2014 (Not All Sessions Included)

Daniel and Brian had a year of manic episodes that brought some small but very significant steps forward, based on the harm-reduction mindset (vs. AA steps). It was a time when both Brian and I told Daniel that we working with him by choice—and neither of us have any thought of pulling away.

February 2, 2014: The recent death of actor Phillip Seymour Hoffman brings up "using" memories for Daniel, in particular, when he used heroin a year ago and got so physically sick afterward. Daniel says that reaching out to me or one of his doctors is NOT like calling a sponsor, and therefore more acceptable to him.

February 20, 2014: Daniel had a "revelation," and says that "using" thoughts often occur when he eats a lot of junk food and smokes cigarettes. When he realized this, he increased his Seroquel from 400mg to 600mg, and this made him feel that he had a way of dealing with the urges in a productive way

March 13, 2014: Daniel is feeling manic and wanting to use. I ask him if there is a time he would need to be hospitalized. He said he would trust me, Brian, and Dr. Grant if we had to make this decision. Daniel needs to tell someone he has been using, but confines this to the meth group, and Patrick, Brian, and me. Telling anyone else is just not helpful. Daniel says he can't "be myself emotionally in my own house." Not good!

April 7, 2014: People who don't know Daniel very well can't tell the difference between his normally ebullient personality and mania. Luckily, the people closest to him, for sure Brian and I, can distinguish this. There is an abrupt seasonal change, and this brings on some bouts of rage and a foul mood. This passes and Daniel announces he has "called a truce with God and will just allow faith in my life."

June 6, 2014: We discussed what I learned when I heard a presentation from psychiatrist, Sally Satel, M.D., in New York City. Her belief is that neuroscience is a helpful, but limited, way to explain the many factors that shape our identity and our behavior. To believe otherwise is "misguided and potentially dangerous." She co-authored *BRAINWASHED: The Seductive Appeal of Mindless Neuroscience* with Scott O. Lilientfeld. (Published by Basic Books, 2013.)

July 3, 2014: Current relapse of cycling bipolar symptoms came on after not using for two months. We are not totally surprised, since this was right after vacation ended after not using. Ironic that now Daniel says this was the best vacation ever. Daniel was almost despondent, and for some reason, does NOT want to admit that his serious relapses are symptoms of his bipolar diagnosis. Daniel says this is because he doesn't want Brian to think of him as "my crazy husband." Brian assures Daniel he doesn't feel this way, and he worries that he puts too much pressure on Daniel (haven't a clue what he is talking about), but Brian just wants to make sure nothing he is doing is contributing to the relapses or the mania.

July 10, 2014: Daniel is frustrated because of a computer glitch and losing some files of his writing. He shares lots of his ideas about future writing/editing process (Brian will gladly help) and "lessons learned." Daniel agrees to write more about depression and mania, saying it's easier for him to accept depression than mania. For him, mania almost always results in self-harm and horrifyingly, turns into "this is what I deserve." Every time the idea of moving from Minnesota comes up, Brian is much more ready to do this than Daniel. Daniel continues to say he won't leave until the book is finished and how painful it will be to leave therapy and his support system, especially when he has his "episodes." He said, "I'm tired of being the one in this relationship who struggles the most."

July 17, 3014: Advised Daniel to call Dr. Grant today. He is eating poorly, and this may be the start of a self-destructive cycle. He is experiencing unhealthy fantasies about having sex outside the relationship. We agree there is no need to share this with Brian because he has no intention of acting on this. Daniel said that when he feels mania approaching, he will start hiding from people close to him. He fears that they will no longer accept him, and start seeing him as "crazy."

July 25, 2014: Dr. Grant tells Daniel that only about one percent of the population has Daniel's type of bipolar disorder. Changed Daniel's prescription of Propanonol to Neurontin (gabapentin) because it works more directly on the brain. He also doubled the Saphris. Daniel is supposed to call Dr. Grant in one week and may be switched from Effexor to Wellbutrin. Dr. Grant tells Daniel that occasional marijuana use is okay for anxiety.

August 4, 2014: Daniel continues to struggle with eating in a healthy way. Probably as a result of his medications, because he says he is ALWAYS hungry, can eat large amounts of food, but then feels physically ill.

August 13, 2014: Another joint session. Daniel *used* for two hours over the weekend, and finally told Brian on Sunday. Daniel said he was sweating profusely and chewed on his tongue!

Brian said the hardest part for him was being lied to for three days. As usual, Brian feels like it's his fault somehow, and he wants to behave in a way that would reduce Daniel's harm when he uses. Painful session: Daniel says he doesn't tell Brian because he is "protecting him and doesn't want him to sink to his level." Brian says, "I'm not good enough for you. I could never relapse (on alcohol) and keep pulling myself back together." Although a very tough weekend, here was a major change: Daniel used, but then went home! Brian did not have to start looking for him. The essence of harm-reduction theory is that small changes are still changes, and are significant.

September 4, 2014: Daniel is the only one in his family who "wears his heart on his sleeve." We believe that Daniel is THE family member who expresses emotion more than any other. This is a heavy duty, and not always met with acceptance or understood by the family. Not surprising… we are just beginning to understand it ourselves.

November 11, 2014: Having his job has made a big difference in his life, and he feels particularly good about paying for his clothing bill himself.

December 18, 2014: Had *using* dreams for five days. This is a very common phenomenon among drug users, even if they had not used for many years. Over the weekend, Daniel and another group member went to the aid of another member who was having a serious relapse. Daniel says that seeing this guy so "messed up" was stabilizing for him—and not a trigger.

December 30, 2104: We cautiously celebrate five months with no mania! Daniel says he appreciates:
> The power he has regarding using or not using
> Interaction with friends and family
> Unconditional love of Brian, family, and professionals
> Continuing to understand mania, and "The feelings I have when I'm manic aren't my fault."

Daniel and Brian had a year of manic episodes, worry about finances and worry about possible self-destructive behavior. However their relationship seems stronger that ever and new tools have surfaced to aid in overall health, not the least of which is Daniel's ability to hold down part-time work, which is building his confidence and self-esteem. This seems to open new possibilities for Daniel to have more constructive things in his life to replace some of the destruction that happens during mania.

Chapter 25

Medications for Bipolar Disorder and HIV

Medication is still the most common way to manage the symptoms of bipolar disorder, and for most people who don't have to be subjected to the side effects of changing the natural way their brain and body works, taking medication for the illness often seems like an obvious choice. It is anything but. One of the wisest things my psychiatrist ever told me was, "Daniel, I apologize for the entire scientific community when I acknowledge that what we have to treat bipolar disorder is simply not good enough." He was and remains absolutely correct.

Years of taking psychotropic medications have forever changed the way my liver, pancreas, brain, and other organs work. I have diabetes, non-alcoholic fatty liver disease, metabolic syndrome, excessive water and fat retention, muscle spasms, irritable bowel syndrome, headaches, nausea, excessive drowsiness, a hard time focusing, phantom pain—the list goes on. Yes, all of these issues also have much to do with my diet, exercise, and stress levels. It is a complete picture. The toxicity of taking so many pills has exacerbated and sometimes caused many of these symptoms and co-occurring illnesses. I have days when I feel just fine and function safely, and at other times, I can be so exhausted and foggy I cannot do anything but sleep.

A lot of people feel when they are on psychotropic medication that they experience their own life as a fantasy. Medications can often make one feel like he is not even connected to his body, floating through life in a sort of daze. This is why many people go completely off of their medication, and do so at various times throughout a given year. Sometimes to keep going, it is necessary to reconnect with the reality of one's own self, as opposed to the reality of the world as experienced by someone who doesn't take these medications. It is also a very personal decision to take medication.

For me, at this time in my life, medication makes sense. It helps me stay healthy enough to embrace everything I want to in life. Besides those sleepy days I referred to, as well as the management of my other physical ailments, I find that the medication has helped me to have more of what I want in my life. I used to find it very comical when people would express their disbelief that I used illicit drugs all while condoning the thirty-five prescribed pills I take each day. Yes, medication can for many—but not all people struggling with bipolar disorder—regulate moods and the severity of bipolar symptoms enough to make a difference in quality of life.

This has been true at times; other times it has not been the case. I choose to accept the consequences and side effects, as serious as they are, because overall I benefit more by taking the medications than by not taking them. I do, however, reserve the right to change my mind on this, and reassess it at any time, which I do frequently with my husband and Kathy. We have an agreement: before I stop taking any medication, I will consult with them both. Friends of mine have decided they don't want to take medication for their bipolar disorder. I support them one hundred percent in this matter. Some utilize natural herbs and dietary methods to aid in their symptoms, and others don't use anything, but rather, experience life as their brain naturally interacts with it.

There are also consequences to this lack of treatment. More severe bipolar symptoms, like anxiety, depression, and mania, are often experienced by these people with more severity and more frequently—and other people seem to judge them more harshly for choosing not to take medications. I think someone with bipolar disorder greatly benefits from having a qualified therapist as a part of his healthcare regimen, no matter how he decides to treat or not treat his bipolar disorder. It is vital as a means of understanding one's self throughout fluctuations occurring with or without treatment. It can be a lifeline during extreme episodes, as well as a responsible way to not rely solely on loved ones to help in coping, living, and yes, thriving.

This is based on my experience, and everyone has to decide for himself, but it has saved my life, or made my life much better on many occasions. This has been one of the many ways in which Kathy, using a humanistic-existential form of therapy, has been an absolute godsend in a way cognitive behavioral therapy never would have been.

I own and understand my actions and decisions in a way that has great meaning to the core of who I am. Had we developed lists of goals and used affirmations, I am not sure we would have been able to reach the same state of health as we have.However, while I am entitled to my opinion, I am not entitled to judge someone else's opinions or decisions.

Does this make me right or wrong? It doesn't make me either. It makes me human, and it is part of what my life experience is teaching me. We evolve as a society by having people of different culture and value systems act on their own passions. Now apply the same rules to knowing someone with bipolar disorder. Let's say three people you know and love are diagnosed with this illness. One of these people decides to use western medicine, one decides to use holistic medicine, and the last decides to live with the experience of untreated bipolar disorder. Each of these people will have unique and personal experiences as a direct result of their decision regarding treatment. Who is right, and who is wrong? Who are we to say? How dare we, as people in a free society, decide for someone else what is the right decision. It doesn't mean the affected person has the right to abuse anyone else because of his or her illness.

If you are being used or mistreated by a person's decisions regarding an illness, you are responsible for defining the appropriate boundaries for you, while he is responsible for his behaviors, no matter what is causing them. My husband has a say in how I treat my illness because he will be directly affected by my moods swings—and also by the side effects I experience from taking medication. A friend treats her illness with holistic medicine. Many mutual friends think she is dragging her family into her world of struggle, and those affected people should have more restrictive boundaries with her. That's a respectable opinion, but not supporting her right to make a decision is hurtful and irresponsible. Her husband wants to stand by his vows and accept my friend the way she is, ups and downs, good and bad, so how dare anyone impose their boundaries on him, or their value system on her?

I dare not, and I don't. I know my own boundaries, and I live by them. This doesn't mean that I don't have my own opinions on things; however, I've learned over time where and when it is appropriate to express my opinions. However, one example is a person who is in distress and is a threat to himself or someone else. In this case, professional support is completely warranted. Sometimes someone is very ill and cannot or will not get the help he needs. This is a viable option like the others, except if it endangers anyone. Yes, it's a very difficult process to force treatment on anyone, but if I ever find myself in this situation, I know I have built a network of people who I trust to make the best decisions for me until I am well enough to do so myself.

The bottom line on this subject is that everyone can have an opinion, but unless you are in the situation, and have to make your own choice based on your own experience, you have no right to judge and try to impose on someone else what you think to be right. You do have the right to use your own boundaries with this person. Nobody deserves to be a slave to someone else's behavior. Anytime I hear the national anthem, I stand and hold my hand to my heart because I love my country, and I believe in our ideals even though we struggle with so many different dilemmas. I see it as a way to thank all those who have given so much to defend our freedom. I also fully support the right of people to burn the flag in protest because if we don't allow this freedom of expression, we are not in fact free. These examples show my value system, and how I choose to live. They are not right or wrong, but rather what make sense to me, and helps me live the best life I know how to live.

Chapter 26

Correlation Between What We Put Into Our Body— and How It Will Function

Chemical Health and Marijuana

One of the things that has continued to make a great deal of sense to me about harm reduction is this: each person has to make up his or her own mind on what it means to be chemically healthy. Harm reduction stops relating the word *sober* to the word *abstinence*, and that change, although seemingly small, has made a huge difference for me—and I am certain also for countless others.

    For my entire adult life I have had a relationship with chemicals. This relationship started at the age of eighteen with my first prescribed medication. Since then I have been on a regimen of chemicals/medications prescribed by doctors. Medical doctors prescribed all these pills, with an expectation that I take them all every day. I choose to take the medications because I trust my doctors, and because I have weighed all the options. While pumping my body full of all these chemicals every day is dangerous, and causes countless side effects that I suffer through, the overall aim of taking all of these pills is to improve my core health, and keep me alive as long as possible while helping me function without the debilitating effects I would encounter if I chose not to take these medications.

Here is the breakdown of my daily medications before the healing effects of my weight loss:

- Wellbutrin: 1 pill in the morning for bipolar depression
- Seroquel®: 3 pills at bedtime for mood stability and suppression of bipolar mania
- Saphris®: 4 pills at bedtime for mood stability and suppression of bipolar mania
- Effexor: 2 pills in the morning for bipolar depression
- Neurontin: 1 pill three times daily for chronic anxiety associated with bipolar disorder
- Triumeq: 1 pill in the morning for HIV suppression
- Nexium: 1 pill at bedtime for chronic acid reflux
- Ranitidine: 1 pill at bedtime for chronic acid reflux and other stomach upset
- Metformin: 2 pills at breakfast and 2 pills at dinner for blood sugar control
- Glipizide: 1 pill at breakfast and 1 pill at dinner for blood sugar control
- Lantus®: 1 self-administered shot at bedtime for blood sugar control
- Lopid: 1 pill in the morning and 1 pill at bedtime for high triglycerides
- Lovaza: Prescription omega-3 supplements, 2 in the morning and 2 at bedtime for high triglycerides
- Lisinopril: 1 pill at bedtime for high blood pressure

This list of medications was reduced by eight prescriptions a day after my bariatric surgery. I still take several medications a day to treat the HIV, bipolar disorder, and some of the side effects from those medications like acid reflux, but so many side effects were eliminated by not having to take so many pills all the time. Also, tens of thousands of dollars, most of which has been covered by insurance of some sort, are saved every month as well.

In addition to these prescribed medications, I also use two multivitamins a day, B12 supplement, iron, calcium with vitamin D, and when mania or depression symptoms become med-resistant, marijuana.

NOTE: Openly writing about my marijuana use is not an easy thing to do. I am not embarrassed or ashamed that I use the drug, nor do I think I am doing anything detrimental to my chemical health. In fact, marijuana is one of the only medicines I have used that has worked so effectively, and without any side effects. I do not sit around wasting my life and time being stoned all day, but rather it calms my nerves, eases my mental stress, and reduces the physical symptoms of my chronic anxiety. I discovered the medicinal use of marijuana after having a period of two years where I would have a severe manic episode every two months or so, and would have brief recurrence of meth use during the episode.

While I claim full responsibility for my decision to use every time I have done so, you must try to understand how my brain functions when in full mania. I become wholly obsessed with risk when I am manic. I want to do everything faster, higher, with less protection, and with maximum impact. I function while manic through impulsivity, and have no real filter for assessing the danger of acting on the thoughts that I cannot control. For me, mania is a non-stop craving for overdosing on meth—and being treated degradingly. It is sexual energy that cannot be satiated, and a desire to be hurt physically by others. Is this crazy? No, it is mania. Some people have their mania manifest in other ways, and others have their mania manifest like mine.

I wish I was one of those people who just get creative, and can get through the days and nights of sleeplessness without it affecting their judgment or their thoughts, but alas I am not. For years I struggled to get through these episodes alive, and since I am still here, I can only say that I got lucky.

Severe Manic Episode...

After a few very severe manic episodes in 2013 and 2014, I knew that I had to find some way to curb the mania until it passed—or I was certainly going to overdose. I would shoot up a large amount of meth at once, and then put myself in dangerous situations with strangers where I was all but passed out from the drugs. If there were other drugs available, I would take them, too. I remember once I had what is referred to as a "speedball," which is heroin and meth mixed and injected at the same time from the same syringe. I used ketamine, a tranquilizer, and GHB, commonly referred to as the date rape drug.

These occurrences of use and mania were awful because I felt and acted like my life was absolute garbage. I would worry my husband to death, and I did not have answers as to how or why I would do this to myself, to us. These using episodes lasted about 24–48 hours, but would take weeks for recovery. I was fortunate enough to have the love, support and understanding of my amazing husband, my medical professionals, and good friends. I made it out of these episodes, and learned a lot about my changing manic states, and how I could manage the dangerous times in the future without engaging in any harmful behavior.

It is truly a phenomenon that ninety-nine percent of my life is lived according to my strong value system and with great integrity—and no desire to use. It is the one percent that gets me into so much trouble, and after having these recurrences of use, I decided that I was open to trying *anything* to stop them from happening again. That is how the suggestion of using marijuana was born. I was sharing at my weekly harm-reduction support group about my last use of meth. I was so ashamed of what had happened, and terrified that if anyone in my or my husband's family found out, they would certainly start treating me differently. A conversation started in the group about how I could avoid having this problem in the future, a problem, which at worst would kill me, and at best, would destroy my self-esteem and my family. Then a couple of the group members began discussing their relationship with marijuana. They told me about how good it worked for anxiety, and how it slowed everything down in the mind for a while, and about how it posed no threat to them when they used it.

Of course I was terrified that because I was a drug abuser, I would never be able to use this drug medicinally, but as I said, I was desperate and willing to try anything. So, with the help of one of the group members, and the full support of my husband, I bought some marijuana to have on hand in the event of another manic episode. Sure enough, two months or so later I was finding my mind swept away again with thoughts of self-harm, and I was not able to turn off my mind—so I tried the pot. I could not believe how effective it turned out to be. Instead of suffering through several days of not sleeping, thoughts racing, and impulsive decision-making that completely ignored everything sacred to me, I instead found that my mind calmed and slowed, my body became relaxed, and my thoughts turned from self-harm to harmless. I still called my psychiatrist and psychologist to let them know that I was encountering a manic episode. The episode was monitored for a few days in close collaboration with them, some close friends, my husband, and myself. It passed without incident, and I was so relieved.

When it was all over, I was able to put the marijuana away and continue on without any addictive behavior. I am still hyper-vigilant about how and when I use this drug. I have a system of checks and balances set up with people I know and trust who know when I am using this particular drug. For the past year I have been without a major manic episode, my anxiety has been less of an obstruction to my daily life, and I have been more productive and focused. I do not smoke pot every day, but I do find it useful for mood stabilization when needed. I am suffering less, nobody is being hurt by my actions when under the influence of bipolar episodes, and I am able with much greater ease and control to navigate the dark and scary thoughts that come. It doesn't stop the mania or keep it at bay, but it does seem to greatly aid in my ability to navigate the manic episodes with much more safety and efficacy.

I said previously that writing about this is scary, and it has been. I think this is because there is a very lively debate in this country about whether or not marijuana is dangerous. I think I have come to the conclusion that it is not very different from most things like this. It is a personal choice and responsibility. If I am going to include marijuana in my medicine regimen, I need to be sure that my doctors know I am using it, that my husband and I are not in any danger having it around, and that I am using it for the right reasons and in the right amounts. I have done all of these things, and it is working, so at this time, I do not see the harm, and I am comfortable with my decision to include marijuana in the list of other medications that I continue to use to manage my bipolar disorder and other illnesses.

This is yet another way in which harm reduction has allowed me to make better decisions for me and for my overall health. The 12-step model would not consider me "sober" because of this use. This baffles me since I take so many mood-altering chemicals every day—and that is considered acceptable—but this one is seen as a gateway to illicit drug use that is dangerous and out of control. Yes, "control" is funny, since marijuana has helped me gain more control of that small percentage of my behaviors that so disgusted me.

I worry that people are not going to see this drug for what it is to me in my arsenal of meds used to fight bipolar disorder. In writing this I have come to realize that I cannot consider that worry in my decision. I am doing what works for me, and I can live with that. The world is going to come to terms with marijuana, and I have a head start.

Failure of Integrity

My first marriage failing wreaked havoc on my mind for a long time after it happened. I remember feeling like a complete failure. My first husband found out about my drug use the week before our wedding, and we had a $45,000 wedding already planned and paid for. That is why I think we both went through with the wedding itself. We had already been married privately the week previous in Massachusetts, which at the time was the only state with legalized marriage for same sex couples, and at that time, I had not disclosed my drug use and infidelity to him.

This true failure of integrity is one of my biggest regrets in life. The 300-person invite list was all ready for that wedding, and so we went through with it, but the marriage never really had a chance. I think the size of that wedding, and how public it was, made the failure of the marriage that much more complicated and psychologically damaging. When you stand up in front of everyone you know and love, and make a commitment like marriage and then fail at it, there is a price. For me the whole thing was traumatic, and I swore in my heart of hearts that I would never marry again. I wanted to have a partner in life, but I had no confidence in my ability to maintain a relationship at the level of marriage.

The Pain of Being Bipolar

Bipolar depression is very painful—with a sadness that runs so deep, and spreads so far, taking over the mind, heart, and spirit as it deepens. It often feels like your mind is in a room that keeps getting darker and darker, and no matter how many candles you light, you just cannot seem to see the light of hope. Despair is a terrifying state of mind that fills the mind with lies and self-loathing. It is strong, overwhelming, and nearly impossible to manage.

When you have a brain that is attacked by the army of depression, it can and does usually seem to be unconquerable. Depression comes full of lies—lies about yourself and that you are no good and do not deserve anybody's love. These lies tell you that there is no solution to the problems in your life, and that you should be afraid of everything. Lies and fear and sadness. It is stronger than you can possibly realize unless you have actually experienced it.

Unfortunately this fact is often what makes it so confusing for the people who love the depressed person. There is no snapping out of it, and nothing anyone can do can make it just go away. I have found one weapon that is actually quite strong as well: *attitude.* I want to make it very clear that I do not always succeed at keeping a positive attitude. Sometimes even the most positive of people are taken down by the symptoms of depression. The world can seem so bleak. For me the trick tends to be whether I know my emotional state well enough to be able to latch onto hope and positive energy during moments when the depression loosens its grip a little. If I am having a really bad day I have to try to be aware of anything good around me. Sometimes I might hear a song I love that brings back a memory, and I latch onto that. Sometimes I might get an unexpected card in the mail, or someone might let me go ahead in a shopping line. It really can be anything good, and a lot of times if I can latch onto that one good thing, I can beat the depression back for a little while, at least enough to find solace, hope, and rest.

This happened one weekend. After about a week of having no desire to live or do anything, I was able to latch onto something my husband said to me. Depression spreads like a fire. The oxygen it breathes is the lies it tells your brain—that you are stupid, ugly, fat, worthless, hopeless, helpless, subhuman, damned, pathetic, and undeserving of love. When you take away the lies, when someone shows you love in that time of darkness, many times you can suck in that love and snuff out the lies, even if only for a little while. That little bit of hope and light sometimes can give you a chance to not feel so burned by depression's fire.

When you are depressed, you do not need people to cheer you up or make you happy, you just need to be loved because depression is a void where self-loathing and self-hatred overwhelm you.

I was able to latch onto my husband's love, and I managed to have 48 hours free of the depression. Those two days gave me the strength to keep fighting it when the depression returned. The point is while we cannot just make depression go away, we can often but not always, decide to engage in the world anyway, and give and receive as much love as possible. Attitude and outlook breed more of whatever they are—negative breeds negative, and positive breeds positive. Hate breeds more hate, and hate runs on fear, which is perhaps the most prolific breeder of all. If I give into the fear and let it overwhelm me, I feel despair.

If I allow myself to feel loved and give love, it brings me closer to all the love that surrounds me, in essence it connects me to God. Really depression is like the world we live in. There are those who say the world is full of evil, and give up on humanity, focusing on all that is wrong in this world. Others say "no" to that evil, and instead look at the good things happening around them. These people see hope and goodness all around them, even in the midst of the evil things. Depression comes into your brain with fear, irrational thoughts, and great sadness. I do believe even if depression is not something that we can just overcome, it is something that the person struggling with it can make a choice about—to make it worse or try to hold on to making it better. I often go through several days in the rabbit hole of negativity, but if I hang on, eventually hope bubbles up, and a little bit of hope can go a very long way.

A Definite Correlation

There is a definite correlation between what we put into our bodies and how they will function for us. No need to scientifically prove this because its common sense. Any machine will work better if you take care of it in the recommended way, and for us humans that means a balanced diet, not ingesting unnecessary chemicals, and keeping the body in shape. For most of my life, I have struggled with this concept in a variety of ways. From the time I was a kid, I was always a little bit overweight. It is a common family trait, but it never really became a serious problem until I started taking psychiatric medications. These medications are classically known to cause weight gain by increasing appetite and water retention, and disturbing the body's natural metabolism.

Over the course of the almost twenty years I have been taking these medications, I have lost and gained the same fifty pounds numerous times. New meds would usually start a fluctuation in my weight one way or the other, as well as noticeable shifts in my appetite. To be fair, this is not the only reason I got to be obese. *I spent a lifetime finding comfort in food.* Eating was a way to cope with emotions and fears. For me, nothing was better than a really good sandwich. The more stuff you could put in sub roll, the better. Carbohydrates, sugar, and salt were always my favorite go-to cravings. In a lot of ways, food was as much a drug to me in life as cigarettes or crack or meth. The corporations that control our food supplies understand this, and know that we will crave foods with these components, and keep up the cycle of eating stuff that often does not even qualify as "actual food," as I understand it.

The biggest problem with this fact is that as a person who is prone to extremes and addictive behavior, having to ingest a drug in order to survive, it is fairly likely to keep the cycle of abusing that substance. Unfortunately being overweight always felt to me like I was a failure—but I never saw it the same way in anyone else. I know plenty of people fighting the battle of the bulge, and I have never seen those people as failures or lazy or slothful. But being my own harshest critic, like most people, I saw my being overweight as all of those things, and it did a number on my self-esteem over the years.

Stabilizing My Mood

In the first year I was in Minneapolis, my doctor finally found a medication that really made a difference in the long run with stabilizing my mood—*quetiapine fumerate*, branded as Seroquel®. Seroquel is classified as an antipsychotic medication. In our society, we often equate psychotic with criminal or deeply disturbed behavior and thinking. Psychosis for me happens when I am experiencing a true manic or depressive state. It does not cause me to act criminally, but rather the way my brain functions, the thoughts that I have become so erratic and illogical that it justifies abnormal behaviors.

To clarify, suicide seems a viable and promising option sometimes during my depressions, and I have often made illogical decisions while in states of mania. Things that I never would consider while balanced became chronic thoughts and impulses in my brain when in these altered states. My ability to make healthy and rational decisions becomes impacted. For instance, I make completely different decisions surrounding how I use my money when in different states of mind. When I'm manic, I usually rack up credit card debt, spending money on things I cannot afford. Conversely, when I am depressed, I usually do not have the drive to spend money on anything. I have been known to go into a store in this state of mind for some specific items, and walk out not having bought anything because I could not decide between toothpaste brands, or which kind of toilet paper to buy.

These states are not how I live a large percentage of my life, but they do happen enough for me to have to remain mindful of what my mood state is. The Seroquel has greatly helped me not have so many of these alterations, and thus has helped me not have to live in a state of mind that is constantly causing these psychosis. Seroquel is notorious for causing weight gain. Your appetite on this medication can become insatiable, which was certainly the case for me.

Of course, no medication was ever completely to blame for my weight gain, but it certainly did not help. On top of that, the dose I need to take of this medication for it to be effective is extremely high. Every other antipsychotic that we have tried has not worked well so Seroquel has become, and I anticipate will remain, a part of my medicine regimen for a long time. The weight at some point really spiraled out of my control, and I began to suffer from other weight-related ailments: high blood pressure, diabetes type 2, and even fatty liver disease. After discussing all of my options with all my doctors, I decided to go ahead with weight-loss surgery.

Weight-loss Surgery

In 2015, at 275 pounds, I was at my highest-ever weight…and I finally had enough. I began eating non-processed foods and trying to exercise regularly, and that helped, but only to a point. I would gain and lose 10–15 pounds like a merry-go-round. What I could do on my own was not enough to make a real difference for my health concerns, and I had no faith that even if I could lose the weight, I could keep it off.

I began exploring the option of bariatric surgery with the support of my doctors. For six months I met with a nutritionist, and a team of surgeons developed a path to surgery. The process was extensive, and the requirements to actually be approved for this surgery are extensive. Besides the monthly nutritionist visits, I also had weight-loss requirements. I was told that I had to lose and keep off a certain amount of weight before I could be approved for the surgery, which is true for everyone hoping to have the surgery performed. The reason is to prove there is a fundamental shift in the way that the client manages his own eating habits—and that the change is not just happening surgically. Surgery is only a viable option if there is a shift in the way that you use food. It would be futile to have the surgery performed, only to continue with bad eating habits.

The surgery is not a cure-all. If there is no change in eating habits, the likelihood of long-term success is greatly diminished because while at first there is a much smaller capacity for food intake due to the smaller size of the stomach, over time the stomach can be stretched back out.

My procedure was called a *sleeve gastrostomy*. This operation involved a short hospital stay. The surgeon would do a laparoscopic procedure where he would remove eighty percent or so of my stomach, creating a stomach that was more of a sleeve shape like a banana as opposed to the melon shape of my existing stomach. The surgery would allow me to get full faster, thus requiring significantly fewer calories to get through the day and be satisfied. It is not a quick fix; in fact the process of getting the surgery approved is very hard.

What terrified me most about the entire thing was the idea that I would be drastically reducing the impact of food in my daily life. I have always been overweight, but it got out of control in my thirties. I was never full, or, better put, I was always hungry. I ate frequently for that reason, but I also ate to be social, to cope with emotions, to celebrate life's events, the list goes on. I toiled over the decision, mostly because of my own doubt that I could do what I would have to make the surgery a long-term success, and also because of fear of the unknown.

Unlike the lap band, the sleeve gastrostomy is a permanent fix, although there have been cases when people who returned to overeating after the surgery have stretched their own stomachs back out again, and put the weight back on. I did not want to be one of those people, and I realized that this was totally up to me. If I could make the changes in my habits, I would gain some greater control over my health in many areas. I had to try, and so I went ahead with the surgery. It was one of the smartest decisions I have ever made. After the surgery, the weight began to peel off me like layers of an onion. Almost instantly my diabetes medications were discontinued, and my blood sugars returned to completely normal, and stayed there.

Of course the diabetes could return some day, and I will be vigilant about that, but at this time my body was taking care of itself again without any of the four medications used to control the blood sugar. My liver, which always provided me with an ache, sort of like a stitch that runners get, must have been immediately relieved by the rapid weight loss as the pain subsided. Here again I have to be vigilant. I still have NASH, but am assured I can greatly improve the odds that it will not get worse if I lose more weight and keep it off.

After all was said and done, I ended up losing 115 pounds in all. My energy level, which has been very low for several years, has greatly improved. I am finally able to get through my days without a nap, whereas I used to sleep several hours during the day every day. My blood pressure, which at one point was so high it was affecting my kidney function, returned to completely normal levels. As more and more positive effects happened, I found myself feeling less and less bondage around food. I know that I can still enjoy all the foods I loved before—but I can eat smarter, healthier and in amounts that won't jeopardize my health. I have no desire to return to the fast foods or the binge eating. It is not always easy, but I have the confidence to do what I need in order to avoid the type of eating that was, quite frankly, killing me.

Losing 115 pounds is an amazing gift, and while I look a lot better and feel a lot better about my weight, I am still struggling with what I put into my body. Some days I don't want to eat anything, and on other days I eat snacks throughout the day instead of eating actual meals. I do not get enough protein, which is very important because the body without protein breaks down muscle tissue, and the biggest muscle in the body is the heart, so being protein deficient is a very real problem. Alas, Rome was not built in a day, so all I can do is keep trying to eat right, keep a clean and healthy body, and accept that harm reduction applies in this area, too.

As the weight came off, the diseases started to correct themselves. I am no longer diabetic, my liver has returned to a normal size, and does not ache anymore. My body used to run hot all the time. My poor husband suffered through many a Minnesota winter night with the window open because I was always hot, but these days I always seem to be cold. The food was killing me, now it's not—and I have likely spared myself many possible weight-related illnesses, and even extended my life span.

Moderation, oh how I battle with thee.

Attending Kathy's Group Therapy Sessions

Every Wednesday afternoon for about three years (2013–2016) until I moved back East, I had been attending a group therapy session that is run by Kathy Vader. The group regularly includes the same three to seven men week in and week out. All of us are over thirty years old, and all of us are former crystal meth users. It is in this group where I have been able to work out many of my concerns regarding what we refer to as the *post-meth effect*. This term relates to the many lagging biological and psychological challenges that exist for a former meth addict. We also address recurrence-of-use issues, should any of our group members experience one, and we support the overall mental health of one another as we make strides in our lives free from crystal meth.

Of course that is a lot to cover in a 90-minute period once per week, but what ends up happening the most is we have tremendous discussions about a myriad of issues. These issues range from living with mental health and physical diagnoses, to relationships and sex, to just making it through the hard days. We also try to keep a positive focus in the group discussion. We share our challenges and the negative things happening in our lives, but we also make sure that when we discuss these issues, we look as a group at ways that each individual can improve his own situation and conquer his own challenges.

One of my favorite aspects is that it is a discussion group. We are all encouraged to participate in talking about one another's topics, and by doing so, we are able to see several perspectives on the same issue. Having many points of view is so helpful because we all do things in different ways, and when there is a problem with the way one of us is doing something, having others to bounce ideas off of is productive and helpful. One of the topics we discuss most frequently is what we have termed the *post-meth effect*.

Crystal meth can affect mood stability for years after use. Feelings of fatigue, depression, hopelessness, restlessness, and anxiety can and do occur at random times, especially in the first two years after the last use. This has proven to be very confusing for me as I already struggle with the mood fluctuations of bipolar disorder. I am constantly on the lookout for changes in my mood and for increased intensity of feelings as a warning of possible mania or depression. Sometimes I can have these fluctuations but they have nothing to do with bipolar disorder, and everything to do with the post-meth effect. The farther away I am from my last use, the less frequent these fluctuations occur.

I have discovered great support from the group of guys through all of these symptoms. I am able to share my feelings in great detail, and relate to the others in the group who have experienced the same feelings. We all show up as a united front, and help each other get through the challenging post-meth effects and to the other side. This is a good time to point out one of the things that I think both harm-reduction and 12 step-models of recovery do very well. Having a support system of people who have been through the same struggles as you is absolutely the best weapon in the arsenal for fighting addiction to all substances and behaviors. Being able to speak openly about the day-to-day challenges takes the power away from those things, and puts it back into perspective, enabling the person struggling to find new approaches to not using.

The guys in our harm-reduction group keep connected outside of the group, and are always available to talk to each other when we are not at group. Many 12-step groups have what they call fellowship, which means people get together after the meetings for coffee or a meal. It is this connection with other people that makes such a huge difference in the ability of a person with an addictive mind to choose other people instead of their substance of choice. These types of connection occur everywhere in the fabric of our lives. Some people find it in their own families, some in church communities or work communities. Of course any group is only effective if you can trust the people in it, and feel comfortable enough to open up about your life.

We are all made stronger by connections with other people, especially when we can talk out the challenges of our lives with trusted friends.

Chapter 27

"Living" on Welfare Payments

Sometimes I overhear a conversation, or read some post on Facebook about someone receiving "welfare." Everyone seems to be highly opinionated on this topic. Many believe anyone who is receiving state aid should be treated like a second-class citizen. The horrible word "handout" gets thrown around. Immediately having the classification of "government help" is riddled with shame. It paints the earliest part of a picture—anyone who is receiving this type of help is lazy, greedy, unproductive, and in some way damaged.

This stereotype infuriates me, and I have a right to be upset because I received state help for a few years while I waited for the long- and even-more humiliating process of getting approved for Social Security disability benefits. I am a hard worker, a man who pays his taxes and tries to be productive—a man who takes pride in coming to the end of the day and knowing I have done something to make my world around me a better place. Someone I know had posted about welfare and drug testing on Facebook. His post said those who are crying about the unconstitutionality of drug testing people receiving state aid are bleeding-heart liberals who are supporting drug users spending government tax dollars to fuel their habit. The point of this post was to get as many people to share it as possible.

Immediately I wanted to respond with a scathing review of this post, but over the years of therapy I have learned one very valuable lesson—to think and breathe before I act, and especially before I react to something bothering me a lot. I realized I could go off on a tangent and spew my anger, but it would make me no better than the people who were insensitive enough to post it.

This is not to say that I won't argue my point or be an activist; quite the contrary is true. However, there is a time and a place for everything, and this was not it. Relating my experiences seems a much better way to explain the truth about welfare. When I received aid from the State of Minnesota, I was unable to work due to my severe and mismanaged bipolar disorder. The mismanagement started with the poor quality of healthcare I received for years from my own psychiatrist on the East Coast, and was compounded by my own ignorance. Eventually I gave up on psychiatry, and tried to control my illness with illicit drugs instead of pharmaceutical ones.

By the time I arrived in Minnesota at age 28, I was not only psychologically damaged, but also biochemically. This was in part because of my illicit drug use, for which I take full responsibility, and also in part due to a healthcare system that's so broken and ineffective it often creates exactly what it is supposed to treat. After a decade and three different psychiatrists, I found one who had the insight, experience, and determination, combined with the knowledge and preparedness to treat my bipolar disorder appropriately. As I wrote earlier, so great was this discovery of a capable psychiatrist that when he moved his practice to another state, I followed him there as a patient. How can we expect people to be able to cope with their mental health concerns, or any medical concerns, when we live in a country that's not doing a good enough job preparing and producing quality care.

I am not saying healthcare workers are unqualified, I am saying *the focus is on money over actual healthcare*, and people are slipping through the cracks with devastating results. Welfare enabled me to get health benefits, which paid for me to finally see a quality doctor. Although I had relapses during the time I was on government assistance, I was not using those payments to buy illicit drugs. It was helping me to help myself. I feel that getting this assistance and its benefits when I really needed it helped me not only to get healthy enough to get through it, but also enabled me to give back to my community far more than I was given. People have this idea that if someone has an addiction, and has a recurrence of use, this person is a loser, not a fighter. Every time I relapsed, I rallied so deep from inside of me to recover, but was met with the shame of a society that has not as a whole truly come to understand how complicated having an addiction is.

Here's what I did with my welfare money:

- First off, you have to know how much I received in benefits. The majority of what I received was devoted to healthcare coverage. This coverage was only available to me as long as my income was far below the poverty line. Since it was, I received limited medical benefits and $203 per month.
- My rent cost $550 a month, and I survived because my parents were generous enough to share the cost with me while I tried to fight for my health, and in fact, for my life.
- The $203 stipend was used for a bus pass and as my food budget.
- A bus pass cost $82 a month in Minneapolis.
- This left $121 to use as a food budget for the month.

I've read that fewer than two percent of all people receiving government aid spend their money on drugs. In the states where they have done drug tests on those on the welfare program, it has worsened the situation for every person who tested positive, even if they had only a one-time recurrence of their drug use. More money is spent on this testing than is saved by kicking those who test positive off of benefits.

If you still think welfare is a handout, try to live on it.

The person who posted this on Facebook is a functioning alcoholic who is blessed to have a secure, steady job. He cannot be fired without extreme cause, but he is tired of paying into welfare—and I believe it is because he doesn't have the understanding of what it is. My state benefits were limited, and in fact, when they expired, the only reason I was able to keep my health insurance was because I was HIV-positive, and the state had special provisions for people living with certain life-threatening illnesses.

It became obvious to me sometime in that first year of therapy in 2008 that I was going have to think outside the box about how I could support myself financially moving forward. I was very blessed to have parents that were understanding about the severity of my bipolar disorder and the instability it caused in me—which prevented me from holding onto a steady job. Far too many days I could not get out of bed, or I would have panic attack after panic attack.

I had worked for many years as a certified nursing assistant before coming to Minnesota. I had been successful working in home health care, hospital care, and group home settings. I liked this job, and I was good at it. That first summer in Minneapolis I managed to land a job at a local hospital as a nursing assistant. I made it through the orientation period and two full shifts before I had to call in sick for a week because of crippling depression. It was obvious that my symptoms had simply become too severe for me to continue working at this time. My parents understood and continued to help me financially, but they were not going to be able to support me for too long.

At the time I was receiving assistance from the county of $203 a month, but that was not enough to live on. After a lot of thought, prayer, and discussion with my psychiatrist, psychologist, and case manager, I decided to go ahead and apply for Social Security Disability Insurance (SSDI) benefits. I had no idea how hard it was going to be to get approved for these benefits.

The first application was submitted, and after several weeks of waiting, I received a letter stating that my application had been denied. It is common knowledge that the vast majority of first-time applications are dismissed out of hand. Once this happened, it became obvious to me that I was going to need a lawyer to help me get my benefits. I was extremely fortunate to have access to a lawyer who worked with the Minnesota AIDS project and their clients.

Once again, here is an example of how being HIV-positive made all the difference in being able to access benefits. I mention this because it highlights how broken our system is with not enough help available to the multitudes of people who are desperately in need of it. In any event, I was able to use this attorney, and I would not be responsible for any payment until my case was settled, and even then I would have to pay only a small percentage of my benefit award in the event that I would win my case.

We filed our appeal with Social Security, and over the next 18 months, jumped through lots of hoops to get a hearing. I had to release all my medical records, not only for bipolar disorder, but also for HIV and general health. Even though I had documentation of my disability from my own psychiatrist and psychologist, I was sent to a psychiatrist who was paid by the government to assess my bipolar diagnosis. After a ten-minute visit with him, he filed a report with Social Security stating that he did not believe I was disabled, and that my bipolar disorder was well managed by medication. Once again I was denied benefits, and had to go through the process of appealing another time.

Weeks had dragged into months, and still we were nowhere. When I told my psychiatrist about the visit with the government-paid psychiatrist, he said he thought the other doctor's assessments were criminal, amazed that in ten minutes this doctor could disregard over a decade of documented crippling bipolar symptoms. After this second appeal, I finally received a hearing date with a judge who would make a final determination. Once again all of my medical records were submitted to yet another doctor who would sit on a panel with the judge in making a determination. I never met this doctor until the day of the hearing, and even then we never spoke to each other. He reviewed my medical records privately, and made his suggestion to the judge.

Finally in 2011, I was approved to access my SSDI benefits, which would start immediately. Based on my work history, I would be receiving about $1,050 per month, along with Medicare. I would cease receiving county benefits because I was no longer qualified. Medicare would cost me about $100 a month, and that sum would be taken out of my monthly benefit, leaving me with about $950 a month. Every year I receive about a one percent raise in this sum.

Finally I had the benefits, which made matters much better. I still required family support financially as I could not live on the sum I was making, but over time I was able to stop needing their help. The process of getting my benefits was grueling.

I was constantly under the microscope of those investigating my claim of disability—and there was a lot of red tape. It was definitely worth it in the end, but you must have a strong will to get through the process, and I don't recommend anyone going it alone. Get a good lawyer because you are going to need one in your corner. Of course then I had to deal with the stigma of being on SSDI.

I don't think I ever realized how often the question, "What do you do for work?" is asked in day-to-day life. Every time we meet someone new and get into a conversation, or see someone that we have not in a while, this question seems to pop up. It is not comfortable to say, "Oh, I am on disability." What made matters worse sometimes was the level of disdain people seem to have for people on welfare. I did not make up this illness so I would not have to work, and I certainly am not getting rich on my benefits. I am constantly amazed at how many people think that needing benefits is because of laziness, or because I just want a free ride. It is very hard to live with other people's judgments about this.

Over time I have simply tried to educate people who are interested, and to ignore people who are choosing to be ignorant about others being on disability.

Being on SSDI benefits, you are subject to review usually every three to five years. Your case is reevaluated and your benefits either continue or are terminated. You are allowed to work while on benefits, but there is a limit as to how much you can earn. In 2014, I did go back to work at a local retailer. The job was low-stress, and I enjoyed both the people I worked with and the environment. I was not allowed to earn more than $770 per month. If I earned that sum, it was recorded, and I was allowed nine months at higher earnings than that before benefits would be terminated. As long as I stayed below that figure, my benefits are not affected. This seems perfectly reasonable and necessary to have a cap, but I found that one of the hardest aspects to accept was the limitations of what I could ever earn while on benefits. I know I will not make a lot of money, and that is okay because I am happy and have so many blessings. Someday I hope that I won't need my benefits anymore. I dream of going to school and actually having a career, but this will take time—and it is risky. If I ever go off my benefits and then need them, I would have to go through the entire process again of applying, getting denied, appealing, etc. So, at this time I do not rule out anything. I just keep moving forward as long as things are stable in my mood. I am able to keep up with the cost of living as my husband also has a job. If anything were to happen to him, I am not sure how I would get by, so that is always on my mind.

I no longer worry about what people think of me being on SSDI. Those who know and love me know that it has saved my life. They also know that I worked hard when I could, and will go back to doing just that if I can in the future. I do count my blessings for having the benefits, and I do not take them for granted. The $203 monthly state stipend ended, but the health insurance continued. It took three years from the time I applied for Social Security Disability Insurance (SSDI) to the time I was approved for these benefits. I had paid into the system from the ages of sixteen to twenty-eight, having worked an average of fifty hours a week at my various jobs.

- My monthly benefit started at $1,066 per month plus Medicare, which pays for 80 percent of my healthcare costs. I pay about $100 a month out of my benefit for my continued Medicare coverage
- I have to see a doctor for one illness or another, including but not limited to, non-alcoholic fatty liver disease, HIV, hyperglycemia, hypertension, bipolar disorder, diabetes, kidney breakdown, dental care, and psychologist.
- Per year that's approximately 100 doctor visits. Each time I saw a doctor, I had a $20 copay, which equals approximately $2,000 annually.
- Then there's my medication, which without my insurance would cost me somewhere around $100,000 a year.

- Medicare Part D covered my prescription costs until Brian and I married, at which time his insurance became my coverage, and I dropped Medicare Part D.

I am blessed to have a husband whose benefits extend to me to cover the rest of the costs, but if I lived in a state that doesn't recognize my marriage, or if he goes to work for a company who doesn't want to pay for same-sex couples the way they are legally obligated to for heterosexual couples, I then would not be able to afford my medication. Something happens when you go on disability—you find yourself faced with decisions. It is not a one-time decision, but rather one you have to make day after day.

**The decision is: I am my disability—
or I am deserving of the benefits of my disability,
but don't let it define me.**

This decision is even harder when it comes to mental illness. If a person goes on disability because of some disease visible under a microscope, or because of the loss of a limb, most people's response is that the person is exceptional, strong, and deserving. With mental-health problems, the reaction is different. Instantly the person is met with suspicion and doubt. Imagine this scenario. Perhaps this comes from living in a society that understands the victim mentality to be "normal."

Chapter 28

Importance of Trust and Acceptance in Your Life

We are all born with incredible capacities for trust. Those first moments of life are so fragile, and babies come with a brain that's not educated in the way we think. A newborn cannot speak or ask for what he or she needs, but still a well-cared-for child will get all its needs met by its caregivers. The child in some way knows to trust the world around it, and the people in that world to give him what he needs to survive. He trusts instinctively, living out of pure instinct. He knows somehow to cry when wet or hungry. Somewhere along the way, each and every one of us, all having come from an original instinct to trust, experience what it feels like to be totally dependent on others to have our needs met.

Often this cycle comes to full fruition in the elderly years. As our bodies fail us, we can grow dependent on others to meet our daily needs, having to trust that all our needs will be provided. Unfortunately on both ends of this spectrum, flaws and failures do exist. Babies and our elderly are often let down by those they trust, and thus they pay painful consequences. However, we all experience a moment or many moments in life when we trust without question, even if we cannot remember those moments.

So what about *trust* for all those years in between birth and death? That's as different an experience as there are people to experience it. Some of us trust too easily, while some of us trust too little. As with most things in my life, and I have found my ability to trust and be trusted manifests as extremes. As a child I was fortunate I did not have to worry much about trust. I came from a family with two parents who were and still are married. I was raised in the same home from the time I was born until I left for college. I enjoyed having all of my grandparents and several great grandparents alive for many years, with many of them active in my life. I had a birthday party every year with friends and family, and had a fairly well-established system of rules I understood related to what was and was not appropriate.

I was surrounded by love, and that truly helped me to trust. *Acceptance* was a different matter. For all of my life, my brother and I have been on a journey of mutual acceptance. We had little in common growing up besides being related and growing up in the same house, and while that's important, we have grown into having a mutual respect as adults. However, for most of our formative years this played out as oil and water, and resulted in some incredibly inappropriate fights, both physical and psychological. Neither of us was at fault, but I am sure it affected both of us in ways we still don't even realize today. In any event, this tension we experienced as a result of not understanding one another led us to find a lot of the qualities in other people that we were seeking in a brother. Our friends from these growing-up years are as close as ever. One of our most vital needs in life is of validation. We need to feel acceptable to the world, and those we love in it. I think this need never changes, but it is so strong that we will often change to have our need met.

We have an innate need in life to know we fit in, we belong, and we are not alone.

My two parents brought to the table of parenting their own experiences in life, from their own childhoods, to their value systems developed around their own experiences. At some point I realized that my value system and my beliefs were different from my parents. Not drastically so but in enough important areas that it made a difference in my life. Most people find this to be true; however, I was not strong enough to stand by what I needed in order to tell my parents I was different. I also unfairly judged them as being unable to understand my reality and where I was coming from. In actuality they have stood by me every step of the way, even when they had every reason not to, or when their beliefs and mine differed. As a child who was gay, I was scared of the unknown, and of being different. Instead of being honest about the fact I was attracted to boys as a boy and men as a man, I decided to change myself to fit into the needs I thought I was expected to have. Deep down, I feel my family knew I was gay, but it was not a strong enough realization for anybody to address it. Any suspicions were eliminated when I started lying to avoid the appearance that I was different.

The lying started at the age of nine, and it became compulsive. I would lie about everything, always giving answers to questions I thought they would want, instead of the truth. I lied about my feelings, my desires, and my actions. I brought all of these lies and the deep need to feel acceptable and accepted into all the relationships I had over the years. Doing so led me from one dysfunctional relationship to the next. The cornerstone of my friendships and romantic involvements, although partially based on a real sense of self, were also thwarted with an insincerity that eventually led to collapse. The friendships I have today are different, and I have a few very dear friends who saw through my façade, and have accepted me and stood by me throughout the process of figuring out who I am, and living true to those values. I am forever grateful for these people. They, along with my family, round out my love, life, and support.

It took a lot of destructive relationships to learn how to form a bond based in truth and sincerity, based on me accepting someone else just as they are for who they are, and having the courage to be totally myself and show this person to Brian. This is what Brian and I have built our marriage on, and the rewards are immeasurable. I have come to a place in life, through the lessons of many mistakes, and greatly through the process of therapy, where I am willing to face the world with my true self. *I have found that I fit in by not trying to fit in.* I value honesty as my number one value and ideal. At times, I don't do it perfectly, but as long as I don't let my fears take me over, I find I have great integrity through honesty. My word is something I stand by and value, and right or wrong, it is my word and my sacred bond. What then of other people's word? It is going to happen in every life when others whom we love and trust, and others whom we don't even know, will do us wrong. This attacks our sense of trust, and can over time obliterate our optimistic view of the world. This became a huge part of my experience when I had to start dealing with the medical community.

Kathy's Notes—2015

This is a year where Daniel has more drug use—but also loses weight via having bariatric surgery, which improves his overall health and well-being. Talks starts about moving back east.

January 15, 2015: Daniel went back east to visit family. He says, "Because I'm in a place of peace," the trip was wonderful. Visited his best friend Kate. All family members thought Daniel looked really healthy. He told them he is constant with his work and his personal writing. Although Daniel says he still has thoughts of using (meth), he knows this only brings "false elation." Presently he and Brian are looking forward to a vacation in Cancun in February.

We talked about future therapy direction. (I try to do this periodically with long-term clients.) Should we keep doing what we're doing? Should we go in another direction? Currently Daniel said he was satisfied, but would give this some thought. Daniel may consider bariatric surgery in early fall. His doctors tell him all of his diagnoses will improve if he loses weight. Daniel admits using food as comfort, and that he is often not conscious of what or how much he is eating.

March 4, 2015: Talked mainly about health issues, including weight. Daniel says he will see a nutritionist this week. He did not go to his diabetes appointment, but did say he is taking his insulin.

April 22, 2015: Both Brian and Daniel trying to quit smoking (cigarettes). Not easy for either of them, and both are using e-cigarettes. Daniel says he is experiencing depression, which is very common for him during the change of seasons. Says the first sign is that he is not keeping their apartment clean. Will take extra anti-depressant medication, as approved by Dr. Grant.

May 7, 2015: Friend Patrick is organizing a birthday celebration for Daniel. At meeting with nutritionist, he told her he never feels full (something I have commonly heard from people who struggle with their weight). Daniel is trying to substitute writing for eating.

May 21, 2015: Dr. Grant prescribed Klonodine for excessive sweating. I had heard about this from another client, and it seems to be working well for Daniel. More talk about moving back east to be closer to both Daniel and Brian's families. He says he wants to have bariatric surgery and finish the book before leaving.

June 4, 2015: Moving seems "exciting in a good way." Plans becoming more firm, and Brian and Daniel will visit their families in August and discuss moving back east. Daniel's boss at his job asked him to become supervisor. This will not increase his hours, only his responsibilities, and Daniel says he is ready to take this on, and it will start at end of June.

July 7, 2015: Daniel describes feeling "mildly manic," and his sleep is irregular and he has high anxiety. He is acting impulsively and overeating. Daniel says he is again ANGRY at being bipolar. I decided that this would be a good time to go over issues in his life that often trigger the anxiety he is currently feeling. Daniel said he went to work even when feeling depressed, felt good about this, and that he still did a good job. He is feeling anxious over first meeting with surgeon, worried that post-surgery he will have a new relationship with food, and is not sure about what to expect.

July 21, 2015: Lost ten pounds, which was a requirement before bariatric surgery. He's not impressed with nutritionist because he says she is "non-communicative," and that sure doesn't work with Daniel! Ben, the longest attending member of my meth group, announces that it is time for him to move on. Ben and Daniel have shared so many things—using, non-using, social times, treatment and sober-house living, that this is very hard for Daniel. I encouraged him to write about this, which he is doing.

August 4, 2015: Daniel's discouraged about gaining back the ten pounds he had previously lost. Dr. Grant tells him Seroquel is well known for inhibiting weight loss. When I asked Daniel to describe the symptoms of his current anxiety, he says, "It's like I'm on thin ice. I feel it in my gut, and then my whole body shakes."

August 25, 2015: Their trip home back east was overall positive. Daniel felt he was more quiet than usual, and his family commented on this. He experienced some anxiety on the trip, but when he focused on his breathing, it dissipated. We talked about whether or not Daniel will need a therapist after the move.

August 28, 2015: Daniel told his mother he has always felt the therapy office was his "sacred space." She said she was concerned about the number of medications Daniel was taking, but he assured her he was totally compliant with the amount and frequency that Dr. Grant prescribes. Both Daniel and his mother agreed that they had hurt each other in the past, mainly in trying to understand each other. This began when Daniel was nine, knew he was gay (but didn't have a word for it), felt ashamed, and started lying about this. His mother said she feels Daniel is no longer defensive about any of his issues, that he feels better about himself, and that they were really in a good place. Daniel also feels the relationship is one of mutual respect, love, devotion and acceptance. Both Daniel and his mother do everything they can to understand each other's points of view even when they disagree or believe differently.

October 13, 2015: Daniel's surgery went well, and he can eat only pureéd food and can't drink while eating. He craves solid food but must stick with this regimen for two weeks. Daniel said he is moving toward a conclusion in his writing, and is reviewing all case notes.

December 2, 2015: He thinks his feelings of shame began when he was diagnosed bipolar at 18, and he felt he could not tell his parents how awful he felt. When Daniel doesn't return Brian's calls, Brian's first response is worry, then he gets angry, and he feels like Daniel can't trust him.

December 23, 2015: Daniel likes being a supervisor. This job came along just at the right time for him. Job is very interesting and unique, and has a small but friendly staff. It is busy enough but not stressful. Daniel is outwardly proud when he goes to work, regardless of his present mood.

Kathy's Notes—2016

Daniel and Brian are counting down the time until they move back east to be closer to family and long-time friends. The eight-year therapist/client relationship is coming to an end—and both of us have to face what the reality of this will mean to Daniel—and Brian.

February 12, 2016: Daniel describes his mood as "rapid cycling,"—which means depression and mania cycling within hours of each mood. Specifically he is experiencing racing thoughts, being "on edge," extreme sadness, irritability, trouble thinking, and illogical thinking. Daniel will call Dr. Grant today to see if a medication change is indicated. Dr. Grant always suggests increasing Seroquel when Daniel feels manic. Daniel said he did go to work but thought he might be talking too fast.
NOTE: In Daniel's "normal" state, he is a very hyperactive, energetic person. Too often this can be confused with mania, when in fact, it's just who Daniel is. It's important to see a client for a relatively long period of time so that you can distinguish personality from pathology.

February 16, 2016: Higher dose of Seroquel seems to be working to stabilize Daniel's mood swings. Brian went home to be with his family during his father's hospitalization, and returns home tomorrow. Daniel has lost a total of 100 pounds! His diabetes is in remission and his blood pressure is in the normal range. I keep asking Daniel whether writing our book is stressing him out, and he says, "No!"

March 4, 2016: Seroquel is working well, but Daniel's sleeping is still "off." Brian and Daniel are both "ready to leave."

March 15, 2016: Joint session with Brian and Daniel—and for once it's not as the result of a crisis! Thought it would be fun to have them talk about how their relationship started and other things, specifically:

    What first attracted you to each other?
    What have you learned from this relationship?
    How have you grown?
    What has been the biggest challenge?
    What are you most grateful for?

March 25 and April 5, 2016: These sessions were predominantly talk about specifics of moving, getting an apartment, and Brian's transfer to a job in New Haven, Connecticut.

Last Session—April 18, 2016

Daniel had such a positive experience in his retail gift shop job that he said it was easier now to let go of what he thought would be a career in nursing. Daniel and I discuss need or no need for therapy. He is in such a good place that we both decide to put that off for now.

NOTE: I will still be available via phone or email for periodic check-ins, and we both know we have lots of communication ahead because of our joint book venture. Daniel will essentially have the same professional relationship with me that he has with Dr. Grant, which is an in-person session once or twice a year, and the rest via mail or phone as needed.

Chapter 29

A Move Far Away to "Back Home"

In the fall of 2015, while working on this book, it became apparent that some big changes were coming into my life. Brian and I found ourselves renegotiating where we wanted to live, and the reasons to stay in Minneapolis and put down deeper roots, versus moving back to the East Coast near our families. We had both come out to Minnesota to attend a treatment center, and we stayed to start fresh. After nearly eight years there, we had found each other and established our family. We had met and enjoyed countless people and the relationships with them. We had learned so much from this city, and it had been very good to us.

In the past, that was always the reason for staying, but now we had new things to consider. Our nephews and a niece live in Rhode Island, and we desperately wanted to be a part of their lives in a way that we could not from so far away. We also wanted to be able to really enjoy our adult relationships with our parents as they started to grow older, and to be there for them in the future if they should need any extra assistance in old age.

We felt the change happening before we even discussed it. The pull of moving was affecting both our hearts and minds, and when we finally did talk it through over the course of many months, we decided it was time to put roots down—but do it back near our families. Picking up everything and moving is something we both had done in the past so we knew somewhat to expect, but that did not change the fact that moving is one of the most stressful events in life. The time had come, and we decided a few things were left unfinished that we needed to do before we would start looking for jobs out east.

My Sessions with Kathy

Before we actually moved, I knew it was going to be scary, but it was absolutely necessary. We had to close one chapter and move onto the next one. I became aware of this one day in a session with Kathy. I had alerted her to our plans to move in the next few months, and we were talking about what was next. During the session I expressed to her that I would seek out a new therapist wherever we ended up living, and continue on in therapy. She sort of blew my mind when she shared that she did not think that was something I needed to do. Then she asked me: "Daniel, you did not think you would continue on in therapy forever, did you?" I could only find one answer. "I just assumed I would always need to be working with a therapist to manage my bipolar disorder."

It was in this session that I finally came to realize that I had actually accomplished the goals I had set for myself so many years earlier when I started my journey in therapy. The therapeutic process had helped me discover in myself who I truly am, and what I truly believe in. It had taught me that my mental illness was something I knew how to manage. I know all the signs of a manic or depressive episode, and I am capable of reaching out to the appropriate people needed when one occurs. I am blessed to have a husband who is as knowledgeable and devoted to the subject and my health as I am. I have a family who will provide much-needed support as I adjust to life in a new place close to them. And for the first time, I have no apologies I want to make to anyone, no desire to hurt myself, or make my life more complicated than it has to be.

I am ready. I went home from that session with a sense that blinders had been removed from my eyes. I have done the work, and while of course maintenance will always be needed, I am able to manage my own life and my own decisions with clarity and conviction. I decided that I would continue to meet with Kathy but less frequently. I also decided to stay in our support group, but more as a way to give back than to take.

I could do these things until we move, and then I could leave with a sense of gratitude and grace…and move forward. New dreams are appearing in my heart and mind every day. I have thoughts of returning to school to complete my degree, maintain a career, and maybe even be able to get off of SSDI at some point in the future. I dream of the love and joy that my family gives me. I dream of old friends I can be near again and will carry the friends I have made in Minnesota in my heart always, and keep contact with many of them. I will always be Kathy's friend. Our relationship has already changed so much during the writing of this book, and I am sure it will change again, but I do not have to watch it end. It will grow into something else, which is nice, because not every therapist and client end up in a continued contact relationship post-therapy.

As I look back at the years of work that we have accomplished together in therapy, and look through the ways in which my thinking and behavior changed over the course of those years, I am absolutely humbled and filled with gratitude. I have been most blessed to have the opportunity to take this intense journey. I am one of the lucky ones who has managed to get access to really good care. Kathy and I have explored endless topics over countless hours in an effort to help me understand who I am and how I operate. Doing so has empowered me to make clear choices based on my own value system. It has also taught me how to survive when the darkness comes and I lose control of my thoughts. Kathy never told me what to do, or not to do anything. She had suggestions of things I could do at various times, but mostly we got me to a place where I could see my life as being in my control, even though there are factors over which I have no control.

Kathy's Notes:

On July 20, 2015, and Brian, Daniel, and I met because we are stuck in our writing and need to figure out what to do next. Also in our future is that Daniel and Brian plan to move back east probably within the next six months. What does that mean for us, in particular, for Daniel and me?

Fortunately, I have had five children I have had to send off to school, to college, to married life, and to their homes outside of Minnesota. I say "fortunately," because while this experience is not exactly the same as when clients leave, it does provide a model of how to let people go. When I think of what Daniel and I have been through together, is it sacrilegious, or at least totally inappropriate to think of the marriage vow? "For better or worse (oh yes!), in sickness and in health (yes, again)—'til death do us part?

If that means our relationship/friendship will continue in some form possibly forever, well, I wouldn't be surprised. I have been very close with other clients, and then they move away. With some, I actually get to see them when I visit their cities on vacation, with others I keep in contact by phone and/or email. With some former clients, it may be only sporadic communication, but the therapeutic experience can be so intense and unique, it has the potential of being permanent. Missing Daniel will be inevitable but somehow I am not filled with sadness (at least not yet!) because I know we have a unique bond that may "look different" in the future, but will be intrinsically the same. Don't ask me for the details—its like therapy—I'm not sure where it will lead, but I have faith in the process, and I look forward to the journey ahead.

Since I have my case notes up to April 2016, we decide this may be a good place to stop. While this may seem like a reasonable and rational thing to do, it implies our working together is coming to an end.

Trauma and Chaos

All sorts of different events can trigger a cycle of depression, mania, or rapid cycling. Rapid cycling is a roller coaster of up-and-down moods, sometimes over the period of days, and sometimes over the period of months. Rapid cycling is defined as having four or more episodes of mania and depression in one year. As a matter of fact, I am presently in one of those rapid cycles.

In March of 2016 my father-in-law had to have emergency heart surgery, which was a big turning point for Brian and me. It was so hard to get Brian out to the East Coast to be there with his family, and I could not go along because it was just too expensive, so we spent several days apart under great stress. My father-in-law made it through everything well, but we realized that we had to make a move to be closer to family. We had known that for a couple of years, but it is hard when you decide to make a change, especially one as scary as moving across the country to a new state, community and culture. At some point you just have to make it happen…so that is what we did.

We Have Moved—Summer 2016

We ended up taking a transfer opportunity and found ourselves in the matter of about two months completely disassembling our life in Minnesota and trying to build a new life in New Haven, Connecticut. I was not at all prepared for how traumatic a move like this would be. I was incredibly excited by it, but also terribly sad to leave the people and places that had saved me, and become my life. The move triggered an especially damaging mania that lasted for several weeks, followed by a very deep depression and feelings of hopelessness and uselessness. We chose Connecticut in order to be within driving distance of both of our families, but I am finding what I have to do is to incorporate new relationships with familiar people. I needed to start to utilize family and local friends to help create a new support system and put down roots in the community a little.

Brian Comments, from His Point of View

Like many of you reading this, I am neither formally trained in psychology, nor do I experience the flux and instability of bipolar disorder firsthand. But it is very much a lived experience for me, through my husband, Daniel. His story is my story in so many ways, and now it is yours as well. Watching Daniel navigate his mind and, in the process, produce this very personal book, solidifies my belief that for all the unique circumstances of his/our life and his/our therapeutic journey, he helps chart a universal but ultimately unmappable human condition.

As a lifelong scholar/lover of the "humanities"—arts, histories, literatures, and philosophies that ask what it means to be human and how to be humane—I can speak with some limited authority here. But more importantly, as someone who loves and cares for a person struggling with mental health, I speak to those of you who are reading this, because I know that you, too, love someone like Daniel. We all do. The problem of consciousness—how can I know what someone else is thinking and feeling, or, even more problematically, how can I know what I am thinking and feeling and why?—defines much of what we call art, science, and religion, and for all of our questioning, imagining, experimenting, and soul-searching, it remains an unanswered dilemma. I can never know what it feels like to experience being Daniel, but he has attempted—with rigorous honesty—to pour forth his consciousness onto these pages.

Here I would like to briefly attempt the same—to speak for those of us who live with bipolarity through our loved ones. There's the old allegory of heart and head that applies to our personality types. In our marriage, Daniel plays heart and I am head. He feels, while I think. I am swirling ideas, and he is swirling emotions. For all the love stories in literature, and the poets philosophizing about love, there is always already a failure, a disconnect, and something curiously inscrutable and untranslatable about the experience of loving someone (bipolar or not) that seems magnified when attempting to write about it, but surpassing the shame demands the silent to speak and eventually to sing.

This is my love song: "My name is Daniel, and I am a grateful addict."

I watched him that evening in March of 2009, clad in a tweed newsboy cap and vest, stride to the podium with a jaunty bounce before he uttered those words—which at the time still felt more than enigmatic—an impossible conflation of gratitude and struggle. I was/am also an addict, but only hours removed from rehab this was my first meeting on the outside, in a church basement next door to the sober house I had moved into earlier that morning.

Another happy hipster in Minneapolis, I thought, but something ineffable captivated me and captivates me still. Besides an initial attraction, there was something else. Is it his energy, radiance, aura, or magnetic charisma? I wanted to know about his recovery, and why he felt grateful. I wanted to know him. We exchanged numbers, and later over lunch and a long walk around Lake of the Isles, we told each other our stories. As he dropped me at the sober house, I leaned in to kiss him. Fireworks. Our courtship was based on becoming friends first, and then slowly, maybe more. Neither of us had honestly attempted that model of dating before.

The recovery community did not look kindly on the burgeoning relationship deemed "too soon" by many, and when Daniel soon relapsed, I wondered if they were right. At the same time, my first sponsor also relapsed. Watching how both handled the setback changed my idea of what this journey would become. At the time I was struggling with the steps. Yes, I am an alcoholic, and my life as a graduate student and teacher had become very unmanageable due to my drinking. But the whole higher power restoring me to sanity, and turning my will and life over to a God of my understanding, still seemed not just elusive, but utterly fantastical. Daniel, and my new sponsor, helped open my eyes to grace through imperfection.

The program of AA and working the steps saved my life. And that life was meant to be with Daniel. My higher power materialized for me as uncertainty itself. The liberation felt by declaring, "I don't know,"—comforting in what John Keats termed "negative capability," defined by the poet as "that is when man is capable of being in uncertainties [...] Mysteries, doubts, without any irritable reaching after fact and reason"—became a radical acceptance and profession of faith for me. All this intellectualized babble was important to me at the time because I was trying to translate the message of recovery into the metaphorical language of my academic literary studies (and offer quite a number of critiques along the way), but I am forever grateful for the wisdom, compassion, and love so redolent in the Minneapolis recovery community.

Growing together as a couple we also grew individually, and at times, divergently, in our recovery reboot. But we both took the lessons from Twelve Step and forged our own path. As part of my journey, I vowed that I would strive to live life more poetically. This was and remains a struggle for me. Daniel does it effortlessly. It is part of the blessing of bipolar, and it is also just Daniel's nature. He is charged humanity in the same way that poetry is charged language. And just like poetry, he can be difficult to understand, but very rewarding to unpack and enjoy. A running joke is that Daniel is a man of extremes.

Humor aside, his feelings are extreme not just in mood swings, but more central to his personhood, extreme in depth and breadth. He feels everything, and for everyone, in such overwhelming extremes because of his most amazing qualities: overwhelming empathy and compassion. Deep states of depression, and the even darker manic episodes, are absolute hell for both of us. There's no way around it. I cannot even imagine the suffering he must often endure, and watching him suffer is my worst torture. But early on, I learned that as much as I hope and desire and want to help "heal" the anguish, "fix" the problem, or wave a magic wand and "cure" the disease, I am powerless to do so.

I can love and support and encourage, but I will never remove the pain. Learning this lesson once doesn't mean it's over. Sometimes we get to learn lessons over and over, differently each time. Repetition, with a difference, imitation with innovation, might be the poetics of life. What works for us is a combination of patience, mindfulness of the present moment, extreme honesty and communication, fierce love and devotion, and an appreciation for and an acceptance of balance.

Sometimes this can even cause conflict. We don't have many arguments, but we sometimes over-communicate, or sometimes even fight about communication. But we communicate, and we do it honestly. The search for balance may be a natural spiritual quest for anyone, but for those touched by the extreme pendulum swings of bipolar, it can seem like a holy grail.

Acceptance of the still and silent balance of the moment, of mindfulness, and of learning to "just be" also means acceptance of the same balance in the frightening and baffling swings and extremes. There are challenges to seeing, much less accepting, both in the moment. After one episode, I told Kathy in her office that what appeared to be a major crisis, was simply "what we are dealing with today," which can be hard for Daniel to remember when in the throes of mania or depression. The mantric refrain of "this too shall pass" rings out frequently because even in the deepest darkness, this truth brings illumination. Much of our spiritual growth as individuals and in our marriage has come from not just accepting suffering, but embracing it and celebrating the blessings that can and will arise from it.

Daniel... One year Later After the Move—Summer 2017

The move led to a year of incredible transition for me in every area of my life. The trauma of the move, even though it was the right decision and the right time, led to an almost yearlong depression. Mania crept in from time to time, but mostly I battled despair and homesickness for Minneapolis. During this time I did not know if I was really going to make it or not, and I second-guessed our move almost every day. Eventually I realized that what I needed most was to put down new roots in my new home, and to connect with the community.

I found work at a local Laundromat and cleaners. It is a small business where the employees are all devoted to the business and each other. After several months of working full time, I decided that it was time for me to come off disability. This was a hard choice because it is scary. What happens if I have a relapse of bipolar symptoms that leave me unable to work? Well, I was able to maintain this job without missing any time, considering it was during this intense depression and adjustment.

I have great faith that I am doing the right thing. My self-esteem shot through the roof, and eventually the episode passed and I became stable again. Dr. Grant was there for me every step of the way, and we navigated many med changes over the course of the year to get me through it and back to a place of contentment in my mind. Kathy and I did stay in touch, but I did try to manage without relying heavily on her. I am truly living life by following the guide of my instincts. Both my family and Brian's have given us incredible love and support in helping to adjust to life out here. Being hands-on uncles is an amazing gift. Being with family on holidays and special occasions is something we appreciate so very much. Having healthy and close relationships with my parents, brother, sister-in-law and the kids, as well as my incredible parents-in-law and sisters-in-law, is among the greatest of all my life's blessings.

Old friendships that I had to walk farther away from when I left in 2008 are alive in all new ways. I am not the man who left all those years ago, and neither are the people I love. Getting to know each other as we are these days, on a more frequent basis, is so fun and rewarding.

I miss Kathy terribly, but I have been able to manage on my own because of the years we spent together in therapy. We have and will continue to stay connected in a very special friendship, which is further cemented by the publication of this wonderful book together. We both wrote this with the primary intention of helping others who face similar challenges or love people who do, as well for as the general public and students of psychological healthcare. If even one person is helped by what we have taken the time and effort to compile; then we have succeeded. Also, the therapeutic process continued on in reviewing the story of what happened all these years. It was truly an amazing ride, and it continues on.

Gratitude is the cornerstone of my life, and I am so very grateful for a life that is truly blessed by faith, hope, strength, and most of all, love. It's not been easy and it never will be, but easy is not what I came here for, and my challenges have made me the man I am, and at long last, *I love that man!*

Now That the Work is Done—Kathy Vader

Did I ever wonder if this book would be finished? Sometimes yes, but often no, but several things kept me going. When Daniel and I first met with our editor, Connie Anderson, and told her about our idea for this book, she said, "I have edited a lot of books, and I think this has *real possibilities*—and is needed." Those words were so important to me, and sustained me when my doubts were the greatest.

Another thing that kept me going was *knowing* that this was an important project—not only for me and for Daniel, but for everyone diagnosed with bipolar, HIV, meth dependence, and/or being gay, *but also* for the people in their lives. Daniel and I know there is so much pain and so many challenges, but when we look back on what we have written, the blessings far outweigh the other issues.

I have learned to be discerning when discussing this project with family and friends. Early on in the process when I said something about "writing a book," people would often ask, "When will it be published? And that's before we had even written a word! So I learned to share small bits of information about the book with a select group of people. It was their sincere encouragement and interest that helped me keep writing and editing when it just wasn't fun sometimes.

Honestly, this is difficult to say, but my biggest issue was wondering whether Daniel was really suffering from depression when he would go for periods of time and not write—or was he just procrastinating? As a professional, I surely know that when people are depressed, they barely have the energy to get out of bed, let alone do any serious work. But, on the other hand, Daniel's Myers' Briggs type is ENFP, which is characteristic of people who love to start things, but have great difficulty finishing them.

At this point, I want to say, "Does it really matter?" It's all done! I knew Daniel so well when we started this project, why am I surprised that there were "fits and starts" as we went along. When I became anxious about periods of time and no writing, I would suggest to Connie that she might "nudge" Daniel (how is that for passing the buck?)—and she did so with such respect and support that Daniel would thank her and have a burst of writing.

Right now we can see the light at the end of this writing tunnel. Daniel says that he loves the roller coaster ride of all this, and I must admit, I do too! We have fastened our seat belts and are about to take the last part of this ride.

Thanks to everyone who has been sharing this adventure with us.

Myths/False Beliefs– Kathy's Comments

Being Gay:
It's a choice. Really? Is there a reason anyone would choose a lifestyle that brings alienation, rejection, bullying, and gross misunderstanding? If a person holds this belief, it's good to ask the question: "When did you decide to be a heterosexual?" I've seen literally hundreds of gay/lesbian clients, and what I hear them say most often is: "I always knew."

Being HIV+ (the + Means HIV positive):
No, it doesn't mean the person who contracted HIV is promiscuous. Sexual transmission is only one way to contract the virus. We might think of a young woman who has unprotected sex one time, and becomes pregnant. Yes, it's preventable by practicing safe sex, but human emotions often supersede rational decisions in many areas of our lives. The other HIV issue is that the newer medications are remarkable, and the disease is no longer serious. The truth is that people still die of this disease or illnesses related to *long-term use of these medications*. A compromised immune system leaves the person more susceptible to other opportunistic diseases. No, the crisis is not over! Nor is it a "gay disease."

Unfortunately more women and younger people are becoming infected because they no longer fear the disease, and thus are being diagnosed with HIV/AIDS. Other ways of transmission include sharing of unclean needles, and less commonly, blood transfusions.

Being Bipolar:

I have a very low threshold for boredom, and working with bipolar clients is anything but! I have not seen two people who are bipolar who present in exactly the same way. Mania may manifest itself in excessive spending, gambling, sex, drugs, and even shoplifting. And that list is by no means exhaustive. Some people who are bipolar only experience mild-to-moderate depressive symptoms, while other must be hospitalized to prevent self-harm.

Like HIV, the bipolar medications are excellent, but even the most med-compliant patient will invariably need changes of medication throughout the course of living with the disease. Some bipolar patients actually like the feeling of mania, and thus become reluctant to take the medication. Sadly, most of the people who are bipolar that I see are so self-destructive when they are manic that it is definitely not a fun state to experience.

Often the media will describe a person who has been involved in some crime as being bipolar. This can give the impression that being bipolar and criminal activity is closely related. While I do not know statistics about this, personal experience has led me to believe that a person who is bipolar who is involved in crime is an exception, not the rule. This is yet another stigma the person who's bipolar must live with and try to explain to others.

Important Points to Remember

NOTE: Number indicates page in book where it was written

6

It would take a lot of time and more work that I have thought
I had the capacity to do in therapy to finally come to believe,
in fact, I was not powerless to this illness.

7

Now I get it—
I deserve happiness and compassion.

10

Therapy is a garden where the cultivation of meaning-making
and care of the self can achieve full bloom.

16

One must grieve any loss before accepting
the gift to be gained from it.

24

I had to learn I could find value, and in fact,
God himself in the creation that was me, and
the perspective I chose to take of the world around me.

25

I had felt loved before, but this was perhaps the first time
I had ever felt wholly and completely accepted.

30
I was coping with trauma by making the same decisions—
and expecting different results.

37
Nobody can save an addict who is active in his addiction.
The addicted person needs to want to change, and also needs
to be fortunate enough to have access to available help.

43
Creating a false reality, whether consciously or subconsciously, about
what is really happening, and deflecting ownership
of our own behavior, is often a survival technique.

47
I have never heard anyone say: give me more pain,
more trials and struggles to cope with in my life.

48
What was important, and perhaps the reason why my
addiction did not kill me, was I had to keep showing up and
trying everything I could to truly understand who I really was,
what I believed, and why by being alive, I had purpose.

52
Sober living has almost no regulations,
and it is not working well enough.

81
I believe we are all a part of a greater whole, that the whole
is one of goodness and love, and that pain and suffering
help us to evolve into stronger, greater beings.

86
(Kathy) I remind Daniel that he is a person who has
bipolar disorder, HIV, and chemical dependency issues—
but this is his behavior—not his identity.

87
No matter what else is happening in life, each person
has the ability to choose his or her own perspective.

97
Having a healthy and happy sex life for anyone
at any age is a positive and healthy part of life.

99
I love myself, and I choose to take what I am given in life, and make it
something great. Everyone has the same choice, every single day.

104
I know if I meet someone where he is at,
he is more likely to meet me where I am.

102
(Kathy) It is not at all unusual for undiagnosed bipolar people
to try and regulate their mood swings by self-medicating.

107
I can grow and learn as long as I am willing to keep
working at knowing better…and doing better.

115
I lived most of my life in the past, somehow thinking
I never had a perfectly ideal time in my life.

119

One day we wrote down this agreement.

First, love ourselves.

Second, be open to others and God, and love those gifts.

Third, love one another.

124

Lust and the desire to be completed by a relationship are tricky ideas to navigate because they feel so much like genuine love.

133

The "Bipolar Curse," as I call it, is this. I have to be more in touch with my emotional, physical, spiritual, and psychological self than any other person I meet or know.

133

What a wonderful gift honesty is to the whole world. The more I share about my truth, the more honest everyone is around me.

136

This doubt often led to a type of despair that's always the worst, the feeling that I am, as a whole person, damaged.

148

My days were filled with irrational fears, and the nights were spent feeling tormented by anxiety and depression.

150

Shame is an inner belief that I am not worthy of love, compassion, friendship, benefit of the doubt, trust, and joy.

152

The only way to overcome this shame was to walk through it.

157

Confronting me with reality and truth from a loving and caring place seems to help me start to win back the desire to get stabilized, as well as the realization that I do in fact have value as a person.

179

While sponsorship is often a very beneficial tool, a sponsor all too frequently begins to act as a judge as to what is appropriate and inappropriate, what is ego, and what are values.

180

I feel this is a very destructive concept, because having someone understand himself as defective is very hopeless.

183

If we all could understand what we have done and why we did it, we could assess and correct ways in which we caused destruction and hurt in the world.

185

As they say in the rooms of 12-step, I took what I needed. I left the rest and focused on a more harm-reduction based model of thinking.

195

I have been lying all my life, trying to cover up who I am because of fear and shame. It took a lot to get to a place where I could trust anyone—especially myself.

200

I was surely gay, and in my state of mind, this sin that would send me straight to eternal hell.

202
God could be available to me if I chose to believe in things like mercy, grace, love, tolerance, forgiveness, respect, and the unique expression of God that's in each and every soul in human form.

220
When you are depressed, you do not need people to cheer you up or make you happy, you just need to be loved because depression is a void where self-loathing and self-hatred overwhelm you.

227
We are all made stronger by connection with other people, especially when we can talk out the challenges of life with trusted friends.

231
If you still think welfare is a handout, try to live on it

234
Over time I have simply tried to educate people who are interested, and to ignore people who are choosing to be ignorant about others being on disability.

236
The decision is: I am my disability—or I am deserving of benefits of my disability, but don't let it define me.

238
We have an innate need in life to know we fit in, we belong, and we are not alone.

About the Authors

Kathy Vader received an M.A. in Theology from St. Catherine University and an M.A. in Psychology from St. Mary University. She lives in suburban Minneapolis, Minnesota and has a private practice specializing in work with GLBT adults. Many of her clients are HIV-positive, and have co-occurring diagnoses of chemical abuse (particularly crystal methamphetamine), and mental illness. She is on the Board of Directors of The Aliveness Project, a 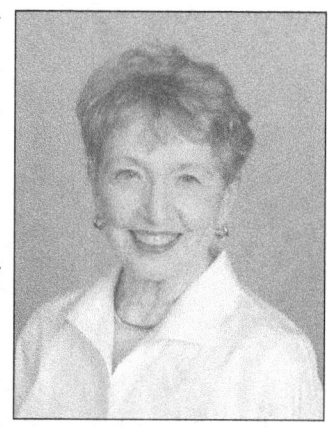 resource center for HIV+ individuals, and provides weekly pro bono therapy for the members.

Daniel Kennedy lives in central Connecticut with his husband, Brian, and their beloved dog, Gerald. He works full time for a local small business. He continues to write and advocate for people affected by addiction, HIV, sexuality, and mental health conditions.

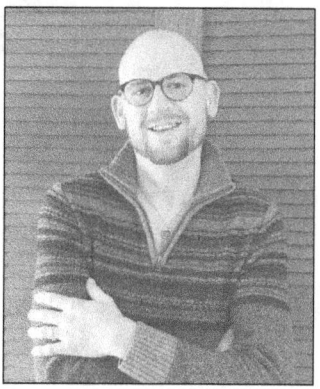

Reading Resource List

Yes, I have read and reread all these books—and recommend them to my clients. They are listed in no particular order of significance.—Kathy Vader

Psychological Treatment of Bipolar Disorder
Edited by Sheri L. Johnson and Robert L. Leahy.

Sheri L. Johnson, PhD, is Associate Professor of Psychology and Psychiatry at the University of Miami. She has conducted research on psychosocial facets of bipolar disorder and her findings have been published in a number of journals, including the *Journal of Abnormal Psychology* and the *American Journal of Psychiatry*.

Robert L. Leahy, PhD, is Director of the American Institute for Cognitive Therapy in New York and Clinical Professor of Psychology in the Department of Psychiatry at Weill Cornell Medical College in New York. His research focuses on individual differences in theory of emotion regulation. Dr. Leahy is Associate Editor of the *International Journal of Cognitive Therapy* and is past president of the Association for Behavioral and Cognitive Therapies, the International Association for Cognitive Psychotherapy, and the Academy of Cognitive Therapy. He is the 2014 recipient of the Aaron T. Beck Award from the Academy of Cognitive Therapy.

This book, by and for scientist-practitioners, combines information about different therapeutic approaches, e.g., psycho-educational, cognitive, family, and interpersonal in combination with the latest pharmacological interventions for the treatment of bipolar disorder. This volume presents a range of effective psychosocial approaches for enhancing medication adherence and improving long-term outcomes in adults and children with bipolar illness. Offering a framework for clinical understanding, and yet packed with readily applicable insights and tools, this is a state-of-the-art resource for students and practitioners.

Inside Rehab: The Surprising Truth About Addiction— and How to Get Help that Works

Anne M. Fletcher, M.S., R.D., is a nationally known, award-winning health and medical writer, speaker, and consultant on the topics of weight management and lifestyle change, as well as treatment and recovery from addiction. The book portrays a "system in crisis" and an alarming discrepancy between the types of treatment employed at many rehab centers—and what research has shown to actually be effective in the treatment of addictions.

Sober for Good: New Solutions for Drinking Problems— Advice from Those Who Have Succeeded

Anne M. Fletcher, M.S., R.D., is a nationally known, award-winning health and medical writer, speaker, and consultant on the topics of weight management and lifestyle change, as well as treatment and recovery from addiction. In this book, Fletcher challenges some long-held assumptions about ways to recover from addiction.

She has researched the myths and contrasted them with the reality about how people can lead chemically healthy lives. She resolved her own drinking problem without Alcoholics Anonymous, and was fascinated by other people who had found alternative methods to stop drinking. She interviewed a range of ex-drinkers, and *Sober for Good* presents their stories: when they started drinking, how much they drank, how it affected their lives, why they decided to stop, what they tried, what finally worked for them, and their perspective now. The stories are compelling on their own, but also included is helpful information about different programs available and relevant research studies.

Harm Reduction: Pragmatic Strategies for Managing High-Risk Behaviors
Gordon Alan Marlatt, Ph.D., (1941–2011) was Professor of Psychology at the University of Washington and Director of the Addictive Behaviors Research Center at that institution. He has written numerous books and articles on aspects of addiction and recovery. This comprehensive volume is both pragmatic and philosophical in its approach to the theory of harm reduction. Included in the book are examples of harm reduction as applied to needle exchange, methadone programs, alcohol and meth addition, and HIV/AIDS prevention campaigns.

Addiction and Change: How Addictions Develop and Addicted People Recover
(The Guilford Substance Abuse Series)
www.amazon.com/Carlo-C.-DiClemente/e/

Carlo C. DiClemente, Ph.D., is Professor and Chair of the Department of Psychology at the University of Maryland, Baltimore County. The author is co-developer of the trans-theoretical model, which incorporates the stages of change into the process of recovery.

This book is for people who are already addicted or at risk, regardless of the specific addictive behavior—and the professional who work with this population.

This Is How: Proven Aid in Overcoming Shyness, Molestation, Fatness, Spinsterhood, Grief, Disease, Lushery, Decrepitude & More. For Young and Old Alike
www.amazon.com/This-How-Molestation-Spinsterhood-Decrepitude-ebook/

Augusten Burroughs, author of the autobiographical works, *Running with Scissors; Dry; Magical Thinking; Possible Side Effects;* and *A Wolf at the Table*, all of which were *New York Times* bestsellers. *Dry*, his memoir of his alcoholism and recovery time series for CBS. Augusten's latest book is called *You Better Not Cry: Stories for Christmas.*

Despite the obvious humor in the author's subtitle statement, this is an incredibly practical and insightful book about Augusten's own battle with addiction—and how what he learned could help others.

An Unquiet Mind: A Memoir of Moods and Madness
Kay Redfield Jamison is a clinical psychologist and author. Her work has centered on bipolar disorder, which she has had since her early adulthood. She holds a post of Professor of Psychiatry at the Johns Hopkins University. Jamison's book examines bipolar disorder from a doctor's perspective, but at the same time, from POV of someone diagnosed with bipolar. So interesting that Dr. Jamison experienced the same extreme highs and lows that challenged so many of her patients.

Gifts Differing: Understanding Personality Type
Isabele Briggs Myers wrote this "bible" of the Myers-Briggs Type Inventory. The author and her mother, Katherine C. Briggs, developed this theory of personality based on Jungian archetypes. The classic work on the sixteen major personality types, as identified in the Myers-Briggs Type Indicator, to show specific personality differences in particular people and give you ways to cope with other people. As Jung points out in *Psychological Types*, humankind is equipped with many ways they might use to provide understanding for themselves and human nature in general.

Please Understand Me: Character and Temperament Types
David Keirsey and Marilyn Bates are authors, trainers of therapists, and diagnosticians of dysfunction at California State University. The book discusses different character and temperament types, which they call "different drummers and different drums." This book challenges the readers to accept people as they are rather than try and change them to be like themselves.

• Daniel's Favorite Books •

The Velvet Rage
Alan Downs, PhD, presents a truly impactful explanation and viewpoint of what it is like, and how it feels to grow up as a gay man in a world developed for straight men. This is a wonderful opportunity to experience the true feelings that so influence the workings of the gay man's point of view.

Evolve Your Brain
Joe Dispenza's book is an excellent way to learn the facts of how our brains are wired and function. It is a lot of information to digest, and the writing can be fairly scientific, but the rewards of understanding how we make connections is truly empowering. Knowing how something is supposed to work makes it a lot more helpful to understand in what ways that something can work as a disorder.

The Chemistry of Joy
Dr. Henry Emmons' book is a wonderful tool in understanding what we eat, and how it affects our mental health and bodily processing capabilities.

Toltec Wisdom Books (of which there are several),
authored by Don Miguel Ruiz, is a series of mindfulness parables and examples of behavior that lead to a deeper sense of self, and how what we think, do, and say, influences the experience we have in our surrounding life and world.

Acknowledgments

Daniel P. Kennedy...

In 1999, I first came up with the idea of writing a book about having bipolar disorder. Realizing that dream some 18 years after it was born could not have ever happened without a multitude of people and experiences, all of which I am eternally grateful for. Please allow me to offer my deepest gratitude to a specific few persons without whom this book could never have happened.

- For my parents, whom I so devoutly love and respect, walking this road with me and teaching me how to survive whatever life deals me with integrity and gratitude.
- For my husband Brian, my rock, my true port in the storm and sun in my fields. Siempre!
- For the GLBT recovery community in Minneapolis, Minnesota, and specifically those of you who have never let me walk through a storm alone and have taught me so much.
- For the Kennedy and Garland families who make me whole, and for all the very special people named in this book and in my heart.
- For Dr. Jon Grant who has brilliantly and gracefully guided my chemical and emotional health for so many years. I offer my eternal and humble gratitude for your unyielding support and superior care.
- For Connie Anderson, editor and book resource (WordsandDeedsInc.com) who took our original ideas and writings and truly helped us transform them into a deeply intimate experience for

those readers that we so hope will be helped by this raw and honest account. *We hit the jackpot* when we turned to you.

Finally and most of all, I dedicate the utmost gratitude, respect, appreciation for, and hats off to Kathy Vader. What I have been able to accomplish has been possible only because of the eight years of her genuine caring and professionalism, as she taught me how to create the life I want—and to find peace through the simple act of *just being*. Thank you for following your instincts with me from our very first meeting. In so many ways, I am alive today only because of things you have said to or observed in me. Thank you for teaching me how to get my balance, own my life, and constantly seek to evolve into a better and better expression of Daniel. If sharing our story can help even one person in a positive way, *it was worth all the effort.*

Kathy Vader...

I must thank and acknowledge the working of the Holy Spirit who has always led me into strange and wondrous places. A perfect example is this book—when Daniel first asked me if I was interested in doing this, I didn't even hesitate to say YES. Really, how crazy was that? I've had moments of doubt, but only momentary, again thanks to a belief that this project needed to be done.

The faith in this book was first supported by my son, Paul, who was the only person that I showed that rough, rough draft to in late 2008. I knew he would be objective, and he said he was drawn into our story from the first paragraph. I won't name all the friends who were instrumental in the completion of this book, because every one of them offered overwhelming support and interest.

Like Daniel, the gay community in Minneapolis has always been my "family." They make me laugh, make me sad, challenge me constantly, and have prodded me to finish this book. And I couldn't let them down.

Daniel...what can I say? We surely have had the roller coaster ride of a lifetime, and I wouldn't have changed a minute of it. Daniel, our editor, Connie, and I surely could not have accomplished this crazy and wonderful work without the strong commitment we had not only to the book, but to each other.

Acknowledgments

Our editor, Connie was always the epitome of patience, knowing that for Daniel and me, this was a "first." Our questions must have seemed simplistic much of the time, but Connie continually encouraged us to ask more questions until we fully understood what we were doing. Above all, Connie's sense of humor calmed me down when I was frustrated or confused about how or what to write next.

Finally, my five grown children never cease to amaze me with their love and knowing what to give me when I need it most—and I needed their support the most when writing this book. And that is what I received from them!

• Addendums for Therapists •

Working With Couples—Primarily Gay Couples

Here is what I have learned...

When I first began working with gay couples, I naively thought it would be exactly the same as working with straight couples. After all, they would have the same problems, like finances, sex, in-laws, children, and day-to-day living challenges. While both gay and straight couples can certainly share these issues, gay couples have additional problems unique to their sexuality.

First of all, society does not universally accept the concept of same-sex unions, especially marriage. So many gay couples face discrimination, even from their own families, because of their sexuality. Thus, the couple may not be welcomed into one or both of the partner's families. In some instances, the accepting family will unconditionally accept the partner whose family is not supportive, and this can help an otherwise painful situation. If neither family is supportive, it is up to the gay couple to find surrogate parents/families to fill this role for them.

Second, two male egos in one house is definitely a different dynamic than a male and a female. It is often not easy for either one to be the "housewife," and they need to figure out a way to divide the household chores that is acceptable to both parties. I've seen lesbian couples who say their greatest stress arises when both are simultaneously experiencing PMS symptoms. As one woman put it, "If you think that's bad, wait until we both hit menopause at the same time." As with gay couples, two women will have to agree on how to divide financial responsibilities, household tasks, and child rearing in a way that is equitable and agreeable to both parties.

My anecdotal, non-researched observation is that same-sex couples seem to be more respectful of each other, even in very tense situations. People think it is funny that I choose to see very few heterosexual couples, but this is my reason—and it certainly does not apply universally. What often happens is that the straight couple will come in, both will be congenial for a few sessions, but when the session becomes difficult, the man will become intimidating and the woman tends to become "victimy."

(I know "victimy" is not a word, but it is the only one I can think of that describes what I'm trying to convey—and can be clearly understood by others.)

This pattern is a difficult one to break for heterosexual couples—even in a therapeutic setting—and leaves me feeling frustrated and ineffectual. Maybe because when relationship therapy is between two same-sex individuals, this dynamic is not often present and therefore provides me, and hopefully the clients, with a more satisfying experience.

Couples Therapy in General

I suppose it is a universal fact that when we look back at how we did therapy in our early days, we cringe at the mistakes we made. One delusion I held early on was that somehow I could—and had to—fix a troubled relationship. Realistically, this makes no sense, especially if a couple had been together two, five, ten, or twenty years, and the relationship had been stormy and near dissolution, how in the world could one person (the therapist) turn this around?

Gradually, I began to realize that the absolute best thing I could do with a troubled couple was to facilitate honest communication. Basically, the less I had to say, the better the session would be. At first the tendency in couples is each one "pleads his/her case" to me, and I would be the "judge" and decide who was right and who was wrong.

What I directed them to do, and do it repeatedly if necessary, was to talk directly to each other as if I wasn't in the room. When couples start doing this, it is absolutely amazing what can occur. For some reason, the safety of the therapy room allows the couple to say things never before expressed. The best thing I can hear in a couple's session is, "I never knew that about you before." And, not unexpectedly, when one person takes a risk of sharing some unknown but significant fact, the other person can do the same. This opens the door for the intimate communication necessary for healing the wounds of the relationship.

Another caveat: *Don't jump in!* By that I mean, let the couple talk, get loud, express anger, and unless they get physical (I've never had this happen, but thought it might a few times!), sit there feeling uncomfortable and see where it leads. Almost without exception, this will end up with the couple "making up," and each taking responsibility for his or her part in the presenting issue. I had one man say after a session like I just described, "Why can we work things out here in your office, but we can't do this at home?" I assured him that they would be able to do this eventually, and they did.

It may be unconventional, but I have done couple counseling in different ways. For example, I have seen one client, another therapist sees the partner, and yet another therapist sees them as a couple. I have also seen each client individually, and then as a couple. Humanistically speaking, I lay out various ways therapy can be done, and let the couple decide how they want to proceed. It may seem unlikely, but I have had many men say they want me to see their partner individually so that I will have a clear picture of each of them. I keep in strict confidentiality anything either of the partners say in a session to me, but find often they discuss their sessions together as a couple.

I think I can best summarize my theory about couples' therapy with an example that occurred with Daniel and Brian. This was a particularly painful session following one of Daniel's meth and bipolar episodes. Both Brian and Daniel seemed very fragile and so hurt, and then Brian said, "Daniel, you are *so strong*." Daniel looked very surprised, and asked Brian what he could possibly mean. Brian explained "You keep coming back after each relapse or manic episode. I know I could never do that." Daniel said, "But Brian YOU are the strong one because you have never had even one drink after all I have put you through."

This example validates my belief that it is not my words that are significant in the therapeutic setting. The magic will occur only when a therapist provides such a safe and supportive environment that the couple feels they can be totally honest with each other, and talk about their most sensitive issues.

On Boundaries—and Burnout

This is a subject I have put off writing about because I have some fear of how to address the tricky issue of "boundaries." First of all, this has to be an individual approach. Each therapist must decide what boundaries need to be set with clients, how to impose these boundaries, and then be willing to reassess the issue and make changes if necessary. Different theoretical approaches have different boundary "rules." For example, when you see a picture (or cartoon) of the client lying on a couch staring straight ahead and the therapist in a chair—not looking at the client— but taking notes, you can be sure that is depicting the classic Freudian approach. Eye contact is not made, nothing personal is in the office that can give any hint of the Freudian therapist's life, usually first names are not used and the "client" is called the "patient." Formality and clear boundaries are inherent in the true psychoanalytic approach.

In contrast, the "humanistic" part of humanistic-existential theory implies that the client is treated *as a partner in therapy.* What the client brings to the session is what is addressed at that time. Followers of Carl Rogers believe that "unconditional positive regard" is necessary for therapy to be successful. I have clients who say the best thing about therapy is that they can be totally honest and not feel judged. Carl Rogers believed that positive regard for all feelings and thoughts did not mean acceptance of all behaviors.

I tell clients that my goal is to understand them—not change their behavior—because only by understanding clients can we ever be able to help them. Here are some boundaries that I have set in my practice that work for me:

Set Office Hours—and Do Not Vary from Those Hours.
Early on in my practice when I was trying to attract more clients, I would offer office hours on Saturdays. In theory, people seemed to love that but *in reality,* many people would cancel or be a "no show." Maybe having to

go to therapy on a weekend was not as great as it seemed.

My first session is at 9:30 each day, and I offer 5:30 p.m. sessions three days a week. Clients can reach my office by many bus routes, but it is not handicapped accessible because of the age of the building.

To summarize, decide on a schedule that is workable for you, and stick with it if you possibly can. During the last year, I decided to cut down my hours to 38 in the interest of self-care.

Are you a morning person or an evening person? I prefer not to take a new client at the 5:30 time, because by then I am definitely winding down. Many therapists I know don't start until noon or after, but will take clients up until 8 or 9 pm. Know Thyself! and plan your office hours accordingly.

I check messages and may return calls on the weekends and in the evenings, but no later than 8 p.m. My clients know my schedule, and I am vigilant about returning every email, text and phone call within 24 hours at the latest. They are familiar with off-hour crisis services, and that phone number is on my voice message.

Unless I have lunch plans, I will shut my office door, eat at my desk, and read a little something spiritual, and also a really good fiction book in the time I have. This gives me a brief but perfect escape in the middle of the day. Other options might be walks, meditation, phone chats or catching up on emails. The point is—find a way that works for you to "take care of yourself" if you want to immunize yourself from the "burnout bug." (see last point)

I Choose Not to do Phone or Skype Sessions.
One reason is that confidentiality cannot be ensured with either method, and absolute confidentiality is imperative when doing therapy. If a client moves out of state, either temporarily or permanently, a psychologist cannot practice therapy in a state where she is not licensed. Honestly, the main reason is that I know I can't do my best work unless the client is in front of me. I depend so much on what I see in a person's body language and facial expression, which is obviously missing on the phone.

My Practice Consists Exclusively of People over the Age of Eighteen.
I learned early on in my practice that having children and/or pets in a ses-

sion was a total distraction. My office is not equipped with toys or anything that would occupy children. This may sound harsh to some people, but I need to provide the atmosphere that promotes the most professional and supportive therapy possible.

Handling Missed or Those Late for Appointments.
This issue is one that every psychologist I know struggles with. Here is what currently works for me, at least *most of the time*. If a person is late, I will give him as much time as I can without going into the next client's time slot. With people who are chronically late, I have told them I don't want to waste their therapy time listening to reasons why they are late, and I simply begin therapy as soon as they arrive.

People who miss sessions but do *not* call

are particularly challenging for me. I do let them know I can't tolerate "no shows." If this becomes a chronic issue, I send a letter saying that keeping appointments seems to be a problem, and I would be happy to reschedule when things settle down for them.

Leaving Voice Messages and/or Sending emails.
My clients know that they may leave me a voice mail or email at any time, but I turn off electronic devices after 8 p.m. As said earlier, I am almost obsessive about returning calls and emails within 24 hours.

If a client wants to email about therapeutic issues, I have him sign a release stating that there is no guarantee this mode of communication can be confidential.

I have a few clients who find "journaling" about an issue they are going through very helpful—from both the standpoint of writing it down, and then processing this in their next therapy sessions.

Taking Care of Myself—and Taking Vacations.
Private practice can be a challenge for taking vacations because we don't get "vacation pay." But, it is essential that we get away from our office and our clients as much as we can. I prefer several four-day vacations throughout the year. With that plan, I can feel rested and ready to go back to work.

Preventing "Burnout."
Do you know anyone who has not at one time said they were "burned out"? It seems to be a "human condition" that burnout will occur, whether you work with adults, children (your own or others), animals, bureaucracies, computers, or papers and pencils. I would suspect that social workers, psychologists and anyone who works with mentally ill people on a daily basis feel they have a corner on this "burnout" market.

When I was under supervision while getting my psychology license, my very wise mentor said, "You will never experience burnout if you take care of yourself." I have told that to countless co-workers, peers and interns as a preface to discussing what "take care of yourself" really means. Obviously, this is different for everyone.

Peevishly Perturbing Pet Peeves

I guess I really have two PPPPs: the first is people I hardly know (or even sometimes those I know well) will assume that because I am a psychologist, I would be very interested in *offering free therapy*. When I was still working as a probation officer and had just received my LP, more than one staff member would come into my office and launch into a long story about either their mental health issue or that of family or friend. They would invariably end the conversations with, "What do you think I should do?" This same scenario has also occurred with my hairdresser and people I meet at social events who will say, "Oh, you're a psychologist. I bet you're 'analyzing me!" Actually, nothing could be farther from the truth. Can you imagine a dentist really wanting to look at people's teeth while at a cocktail party? Or a doctor saying "Let me give you a quick physical as long as we're here"? My response to people who ask for therapy outside of the office is, "That sounds like a really serious problem, and one where therapy could be very helpful. You can contact your insurance plan and find a good psychologist." That way the person's problem is taken seriously, but gets you off the hook for pro bono work for which you haven't signed up.

Early on in my practice I read a very wise slogan: "Only do therapy in the office, and in the office only do therapy." The first part of that sentence is directly related to what I have just written: *the office is the official, profes-*

sional and most importantly, confidential place where therapy must take place. This is essential to differentiate therapy from any other casual conversation. Only do therapy in the office? Well, I'm sure I've made a few exceptions. If there are an unusual number of cancellations for the day, I might read my book just a little longer. I believe there is always some work to be done in the office—it may be purging files, writing letters to clients you haven't seen in a while, reading professional journals and books, and even organizing and dusting. Not every hour needs to be billable, but keeping your workspace in the condition that best supports your practice is a valuable way to spend your time.

The second PPPP peeve is lay people and even some professionals who will "diagnose" everyone, from people they barely know to people who are in politics or even celebrities. Those of us who do this as a profession know that diagnosis is not a parlor game or something you can learn from Google…or from observing a few "symptoms." I purposely put symptoms in quotes because symptoms most often can be personality quirks and not pathology. Making an accurate diagnosis takes time and concentration. It cannot be legitimately done without contact and taking the person's history. When I am asked, "Don't you think Peter is bipolar? He has terrible mood swings," I can calmly answer, "I have no idea because he is not my client."

How to Handle a Client's "I Don't Know" Answers

The phrase, "I don't know," can have many subtle meanings. It can mean, for example:

"I really do know the answer, but don't want to talk about it." "You're boring me with your questions, and I'm choosing not to participate." "I'm just not up to thinking too hard about this right now."*But*, it can also mean, "I really don't know."

A book written anonymously in the 14th century, *The Cloud of Unknowing*, suggests that we be strong enough to abandon any idea we might have of God's activities and attributes, but instead accept that we are "unknowing." The author says that in doing this, we then actually might get a glimpse of God's true nature.

If we are "unknowing," it implies that we have the space and capacity to accept whatever is offered to us. Buddhism believes if your cup of tea is full, it cannot accept more tea. Knowing when to validate a true "I-don't-know" statement, and when to probe for more information, is an intuitive process based on just how well you know your client.

If I ask a question like, "Is there any connection between how you handle relationships now and how you grew up?" and the client says, "I don't know," I will often say, "Can you just think about that for a minute and see if you come up with something?"

And about 99 percent of the time, the client will absolutely make a valid connection. If, after the prompt, there is still a block, as the therapist I might offer a few options. This could be stated as, "Some people who have similar family experiences…" I state it this way because it is always best if a client himself can see how his past life affects his current life.

If a client ever says, "I'm not ready to talk about this now," I will always respect this. I believe people do have protective defenses that keep them from disclosing issues that they are not prepared to address. Given time and support, these issues will reappear when the client is ready.

So much of therapy is intuitive, and comes only from experience and trial and error. Patience is a virtue when doing therapy, especially if you are Existential-Humanistic and believe in letting your clients take the lead in improving their own mental health.

The Chicken or the Egg…or, What to "Fix" First: CD, HIV, or MI?

When working with a person who has more than one major diagnosis, people often ask, "What do you treat first?" My answer is "all of the above." I believe in a holistic approach and choose to simultaneously address as many issues as I can. Obviously, clients can't do good therapy if they are high or intoxicated. Conversely, I have had some pretty successful sessions with someone coming down from meth, or having used a minimal amount. However, I found it difficult and even impossible to conduct therapy with someone who is intoxicated. In working with someone with multiple diagnoses (like Daniel who is HIV+, bipolar, gay, and in recovery from crystal meth), I find it useful to see connections among these issues. For example, if Daniel experienced shame from a manic episode, would that trigger a meth relapse? I have never accepted the excuse for "using behavior" as "that was the drunk me or the high me who did that." Rather, I tell my clients: "No, it is YOU, *your shadow side*, certainly, but still YOU. To be emotionally healthy, it is necessary to accept all parts of yourself. That is what constitutes a truly authentic person."

When people are sent to anger management classes, I find that this *can* be a way to interrupt the problematic behavior. But a more integrated approach that is directed toward the causes of the angry behavior takes more time, but yields more long-lasting results. Anger is the "rug," and you need to see what is under that "rug" to fully address the problem. The same holds true for chemical abuse issues—they are symptoms, and the causes need to be discovered and addressed.

When I did my practicum at an adolescent sex offender program, some of the staff felt that the main goal with these youth was to promote empathy for their victims. One of my very wise supervisors at the program believed strongly that unless and until the youth had worked through his or her own abuse—*and felt those feelings*, he or she could never empathize with their victims' pain.

We are all complicated, interesting, and often baffling people—the more we can learn all we can about a person's thoughts, feelings, and desires, the more we might be able to help them. Again, this takes time and patience, but has the best chance of producing a healthy and whole person.

List of Prescription Drugs/Brand Names

Venlafaxine is *Effexor*

Quetiapine fumerate is *Seroquel*®

Propranolol—Brand names: *Hemangeol, Inderal LA, Inderal XL, InnoPran XL, Inderal*

Gabapentin is *Neurontin*.

Buspirone is *Buspar*.

Omeprazole is *Prilosec*.

Clonzzepam is *Klonapin*

Aenapine is *Saphris*®

Bupropion is *Wellbutrin*

Abacavir, dolutegravir, and lamivudine combined is T*riumeq*®

Escomprazole is *Nexium*

Ranitidine is *Zantac*®

Metformin is *Glumetza, Glucophage, and Fortamet*

Glipizide is *Glucotrol*

Insulin glargine is *Lantus*®

Gemfibrozil is *Lopid*

Omega-3 acid ethyl ester is *Lovaza*

Lisinopril is *Zestril or Prinivil*

Aripiprazole is *Abilify*®

www.ingramcontent.com/pod-product-compliance
Lightning Source LLC
Chambersburg PA
CBHW071600080526
44588CB00010B/969